Natural Remedies For

Pigs

Mark Gilberd

Homoeopath, Medical Herbalist and Iridologist

Index

How to Make Poultices
Dosage for Forms of Herbal Medicine

Herbal <small>Page 103</small>

Agrimony, Alfalfa, Angelica, Aniseed, Arnica, Astragalus, Barberry, Bear Berry, Black Cohosh Page 106, Blue Flag, Boswella, Broom, Burdock, Buchu, Cayenne, Calendula, Cat Mint, Cats Claw, Celery Seed, Centaury, Chamomile, Chaparral, Chaste Tree, Chickweed Page 111, Cleavers, Coltsfoot, Comfrey, Corn Silk, Cranesbill, Cranberry, Dandelion, Devils Claw Page 114 , Dong Quai, Echinacea, Elecampane, Elder, Eyebright, Fennel, Fenugreek Page 117, Feverfew, Figwort, Fumitory, Garlic, Guaiacum, Gentian Page 120 , Ginger, Gingko Biloba, Ginseng Panax, Ginseng Siberian, Goldenrod, Gravel Root, Grindelia, Hawthorn, Hops, Horehound Page 124, Horse Chestnut, Horseradish, Horsetail, Hypericum, Hyssop, Juniper, Kelp, Lady's Mantle, Lemon Balm Page 127, Licorice, Lime Blossom, Marshmallow, Meadowsweet, Mistletoe, Milk Thistle, Motherwort Page 131, Mullein, Myrrh, Nasturtium, Neem, Nettles, Oats, Parsley, Passion, Flower, PauD'arco, Pennyroyal Plantain Page 136, Peppermint, Poke Root, Raspberry, Red Clover Reshi, Rose Hips, Rosemary, Rue, Sage Page 140, Sarsaparilla, Shitake, Slippery Elm Bark, Shepherds Purse, Skullcap, St John's Wort, Sweet Violets, Senna Pods, Tansy, Tea Tree Oil, Thyme, Valerian, Vervain Page 144, Wild Yam, Willow Bark, Witch Hazel, Withania Wood Betony, Wormwood, Yarrow, Yellow Dock. Yucca

Homoeopathic Supplement <small>Page 148</small>

Symptoms Guide
Disease Nosodes

Materia Medica <small>Page 153</small>

Aconite, Allium Cepa, Ant Tart, Apis, Arnica, Arsenic Album, Belladonna, Bellis Perinnis, Bryonia, Calendula, Cantharis, Carbo Vegetabilis, Causticum, Euphrasia, Hypericum, Ipecac, Kali Bich, Kali Carb, Lachesis, Ledum, Lycopodium, Nat Sulf, Nux Vom, Phosphorus, Pulsatilla, Rhus Tox, Ruta, Silica, Staphysagria, Symphytum, Tarantula Cuba, Urtica Urens.
Vitamin C

Introduction
Welcome to the Animal Natural Remedy Series

These books are an effort to preserve the documentation of Natural Remedies used in the treatment of animals. In the past 100 years most of these treatments have been lost, especially in the treatment of cattle one of our most ancient of farm animals. Other reasons for writing these books is that I hate vet bills and people having to kill their farm animals or pets for economic reasons which I myself have been forced to do in the past on a Goat farm. Originally these books were put together as a field reference for myself, for there is nothing worse than being in a paddock with a sick animal with the farmer, his hands on his hips waiting for you to perform and fix his animal.

Now the books have evolved and have had about 15 years of additions and are offered to you to teach you a new way of thinking. The books have evolved more by my different trainings. As a farmer I learnt to supplement the animals with the deficiencies of the soil so the books always start with the vitamins and minerals and their deficiency symptoms. As an Iridologist I tend to think and work with Body Systems such as The Nervous System or The Digestive System and concentrate on building them up with Nutrition and Herbs. As a Medical Herbalist I am trained to think holistically and design formulas that cover the whole being along with making the formulas easily absorbed. My Homoeopathic training teaches me to pay attention to the mind symptoms and to pay attention to what is really there not what I think is there and to treat and relieve the symptoms of the individual. Homoeopathy also shows how disease taints can be inherited and what to look for and how to treat them but best of all it gives me a special weapon to use when disaster strikes in the form of epidemics, these are called Disease Nosodes which are a preparation made from the disease product so you have a tool to help prevent the spread of disease. The books are set out in such a way as to teach you the correct use of Herbs e.g. thinking in body systems such as the Respiratory System or the Nervous System and in using herbs by their Medical Actions rather then that herb worked well last time. At the end of each system for example The Nervous System we have a section that gives you the common Actions used and needed for that section. Keeping with our example The Nervous System some of our Actions would be Anti-spasmodic, Sedative and Nervine Stimulants. After the explanation of the Action you have a list of herbs that are known to be strong in that action, this gives you more of a selection of herbs then what is mentioned in the text. Next we move on to the Homoeopathic Remedies for the condition which have the details to allow you to select a reasonably similar remedy. Homeopathy sits on a three legged stool. What this means is that if a remedy has at least three symptoms in the same strength as the symptoms you are trying to match then that remedy is a potential cure for your patient or if not cure it will offer the condition relief. The more symptoms you can match to the remedy the better the remedy will work for the rule is likes cure likes not vaguely similar cures. Homoeopathy (homo means same pathy means disease) is a good form of treatment for animals who usually respond to it fairly well and also it is very cheap to use and very easy to medicate unlike the herbs. A lot of effort has been put into the symptom details of the disease as it is very hard trying to diagnose when the animal can't answer your questions, so here you have to be very observant.

If used correctly this book makes you think and act more like a Professional Herbalist and broadens your view on what you are doing. With the Homoeopathics I have only really given you the leading remedies to put you on the right track, it would be worthwhile to invest in a good Materia Medica (Homoeopathic Remedy Reference) such as Boericke's which is one of the best for the Layman.

Main Reference Sources

The original base of the herbs I use were sourced from Juliette de Baïracli Levy's old Herbals, as hers are about the only Animal Herb References that have not been lost in time and they give you a lot of the old ancient herbs that have been used throughout most of history. To these I have added a lot of the more modern Herbs especially those that I use in my own work such as Astragalus and those that will soon be added after using for the first time on animals because there are just no substitutes. A good and recent example is Brahmi which I used in a cat recovering from a stroke because of my previous success in humans with this herb as it is supposed to rewire the brain around the damaged area and in its 3000 years of constant use someone must of used it on an Animal before. There are new herbs coming mainly from the Philippines, Indonesia, India and China but they are still being tried and tested and the average person wouldn't be able to get hold of them but the future looks far brighter than what it was 15 years ago when I started slowly putting this all together. We owe a lot to Juliette de Baïracli Levy for without her all these valuable herbs and how they were used would be lost. She has created a strong foundation that we can now build on.

Juliette de Baïracli Levy (11 November 1912 – 28 May 2009) was an English herbalist and author noted for her pioneering work in holistic veterinary medicine. Born to a wealthy Jewish family (her father was Turkish, her mother Egyptian) and raised in England with chauffeurs, maids, cooks, and gardeners. She knew as a child that she wanted to be a veterinarian. After studying veterinary medicine at the Universities of Manchester and Liverpool for two years she left England to study herbal medicine in Europe, Turkey, North Africa, Israel and Greece, living with gypsies, farmers and livestock breeders and recording their knowledge, especially the Gypsies. "I realized that if I wanted to learn the traditional ways of healing and caring for animals, I had to be where people still lived close to the land and close to their flocks," she says. "From Berbers, Bedouins, nomads, peasants, and gypsies in England, Israel, Greece, Turkey, Mexico, and Austria, I learned herbal knowledge and the simple laws of health and happiness. I never tired of traveling with my Afghan Hounds, always living with and learning from those around me." After living for some time on the Greek island Kythira she then resided in an old age home in Burgdorf, Switzerland leaving the world a better place.

For Homoeopathy my main hero is George Macleod not only for the success had based on his work but in my opinion he is a Homoeopathic Master up there with the greats and I admire his work in the use of Homoeopathic Disease Nosodes. All the high potencies mentioned are his work along with most of the Nosodes for as any trained Homoeopath knows and has had beaten into them during training you don't change the work of the masters. Unfortunately in our fast paced world not many people have time for Homoeopathy but I will say this, in the next Global Pandemic I and my family will be safe because I will make the Disease Nosode of it for I was trained by the Homoeopathic Masters.

George MacLeod (McLeod) (1912 – 1995) MRCVS DVSM Veterinary FF. Hom was a homeopathic vet, President of The British Association of Homeopathic Vets, Veterinary Consultant to The Homeopathic Development Foundation. George MacLeod was a graduate of Glasgow University and was one of the world's foremost authorities on Homeopathic treatment of animals. He was one of the few veterinary surgeons to use Homeopathic medicines wholly and exclusively. He was responsible for keeping Homeopathy available for animals in the UK, almost single-handedly, for the middle part of the 20th Century.

Other animal Homoeopaths sourced are Christopher Day, Edward Ruddock, and John Rush

Animal Natural Remedy Books

Natural Remedies For Cat Diseases
Natural Remedies For Dog Diseases
Natural Remedies For Goat Diseases
Natural Remedies For Sheep Diseases
Natural Remedies For Pig Diseases
Natural Remedies For Cow Diseases
Natural Remedies For Horse Diseases
Natural Remedies For Poultry Diseases

Mark Gilberd
Homoeopath, Iridologist, Medical Herbalist

Pulse and Temperature

Pulse - The average heartbeat of an adult pig is about 55 to 75 beats per minute when awake and 25 beats per minute when resting. Piglets have an average heart rate of 250 beats per minute.

The pulse should be taken with the finger tips at the center of the inside of the hind leg just below the level of the kneecap (stifle).

Respirations - Should be at the rate of 20 to 30 breathes per minute (breathing in and out is 1 breath) in the mature animal but slightly more rapid in young pigs.

Temperature - A pig's average temperature is 102 degrees F, normal range varies from 101.6 degrees to 103.6 degrees. Temperature is taken via rectum.

Gestation Period - 117 days a shorter period signals ill health. A sow should have a minimum of 12 teats. A average sow gives birth to between 6 and 13 piglets in one litter.

Piglets prefer the air temperature to be about 90 degrees F or 32 degrees C.

In one day a **pig grows** in length about 1mm.

A hog eats about 5 pounds of feed per day or almost a ton per year.

A pig matures at between 5 and 7 months of age.

Hogs have a non-ruminate stomach, but prefer to eat energy rich foods like roots and nuts and reject energy poor foods like grass.

Pigs when feeling off color have staring coats (hair stands up instead of lying flat) and their snouts will be dry not moist and shiny.

Notes

Nutrition

Pigs can be friendly and happy creatures if well looked after and if you have spent some time playing with little piglets you would realize that they are also quite intelligent. Pigs are mostly omnivores which means they eat meat as well as plants and they have a high requirement for minerals which is not surprising considering the time spent digging and the amount of earth that would get swallowed.

Because omnivores do not eat much herbage they do not need ruminants like cattle and sheep. The main type of digestion in the pig is enzymatic and takes place in the stomach and small intestine. The saliva of omnivores contains an amylase enzyme so digestion begins as soon as food enters the mouth. Because bacteria only play a small part in a pig's digestion its food must always consist largely of starch, sugar, fat and protein of a high biological standard that can be rendered soluble by the enzymes secreted in the stomach and intestines. Because of the small amount of vitamin synthesis that takes place in omnivores it is essential to receive most of the vitamins required in the food.

With animal vitamin and mineral supplementation the golden rule is to get your soil tested and to see what the deficiencies are in the soil. If your animals are living off what you produce on your land then they will have the same deficiencies as the land and these deficient supplements are the first ones you should think to supplement after checking out what the symptoms of deficiencies in these can do and checking to see if your stock is showing any of the signs. Think about fixing the land as well as the animals. If you find one day that the pigs are looking at you and licking their lips they could have a protein deficiency, think of supplementing fish or meat meal, whey or cod liver oil etc. A lot of the B vitamins, Choline and Iron are found in meat. There is a story of a farmer going home drunk at the turn of the 19th century and the last words to his mates were I got to feed the pigs before I go to bed. He was never seen again. Upon a long and intensive search coat buttons were found in the pig faces.

Pat Coleby in her book Farming Naturally and Organic Animal Care says that soybean meal can deplete iodine. She goes on to say that after 20 years of conventional farming large amounts of seaweed meal, extra copper and zinc as well as dolomite are needed to keep the pigs healthy. She goes on to say that whatever diet is fed to pigs they would benefit from the following additives.

Dolomite - teaspoon per head daily

Seaweed products of some kind.

Sulphur - a tea spoon per head daily

Cod Liver Oil - a tea spoon at least once a week.

If they are totally free range she suggests a salt lick similar to cattle. Sulphur in the diet should stop the skin problems or it could be used externally as a paste mixed with cooking oil.

Fat Deficiency - Signs are hair loss, scaly dermatitis, areas of skin necrosis on the neck and shoulders and a unthrifty appearance in growing pigs. A level of 1 to 1.5% of fat seems ample to supply the essential fatty acids.

Note - In the Mineral and Vitamin Section Herb sources are given. This comes in handy if you know what your own soil is deficient in as you could add some of these herbs to a Herbal formula.

Vitamins and Minerals

Calcium

Function - Assists in the contraction of muscles. Required for blood clotting. Assists in the production of hormones and enzymes. Works with phosphorus and Vitamin D to produce bone, bone is 35 percent calcium.

Sources - Green leafy forage, limestone, oyster shell flower, fish meal, bone meal.

Herb Sources - Alfalfa, Blue Cohosh, Chamomile, Cleavers, Coltsfoot, Cayenne, Comfrey, Dandelion, Kelp, Mistletoe, Meadowsweet, Nettles, Parsley, Plantain, Raspberry, Rose Hips, Shepherds Purse, Yarrow, Yellow Dock.

Deficiencies - Rickets in young, Developmental Orthopaedic Disease, Poor muscle function, Impaired blood clotting, Joint problems and bone weakness, Posterior paralysis.

Phosphorous

Function - Works with calcium for bone growth. Assists in energy metabolism. Makes up 15 percent of bone. Too much phosphorous will reduce the absorption of calcium during digestion.

Sources - Cereals, Lucerne, Fish and meat meals.

Herb Sources - Alfalfa, Anise, Asparagus, Blue Cohosh, Caraway, Cayenne, Chickweed, Calamus, Dandelion, Dill, Fenugreek, Garlic, Golden Rod, Kelp, Licorice, Linseed, Marigold, Meadowsweet, Parsley, Raspberry, Rose Hips, Sunflower, Yellow Dock.

Deficiencies - Overfeeding of phosphorous can lead to lameness, fragile bones, enlargement of the jaw bone, hyperparathyroidism

Magnesium

Function - Required for hemoglobin formation in the blood. Assists in bone formation. Assists in enzyme functions of the body.

Sources - Alfalfa, Clover, Bran, Linseed, Milk.

Herb Sources - Alfalfa, Blue Cohosh, Broom, Carrot leaves,

Cayenne, Dandelion, Hops, Marshmallow, Meadowsweet, Mistletoe, Mullein, Peppermint, Raspberry, Slippery Elm.

Deficiencies - Nervousness and excitability. Increased respiratory rates. Muscle tremors. Aggressiveness and ill temper.

Sulphur

Function - Contains amino acids methionine and cystine. Assists in enzyme and hormone production.

Sources - Protein feeds and Green forage.

Herb Sources - Alfalfa, Burdock, Broom, Calamus, Coltsfoot, Cayenne, Daisy, Eyebright, Fennel, Garlic, kelp, Marigold, Meadowsweet, Mullein, Nettle, Parsley, Plantain, Raspberry, Sage, Shepherds purse, Thyme, Yarrow.

Deficiencies - None recorded but overdosing can lead to loss of weight and appetite, colic, a yellow frothy discharge from the nose and labored breathing.

Sodium Chloride

Function - Maintains the balance of fluids in the cells. Assists in muscle contractions. Removes waste products from the cells. Required in the production of bile. Maintains the health of the nervous system.

Sources - Salt and salt licks. Green forages especially Alfalfa.

Deficiencies - Dehydration, Poor Growth, muscle cramps, Reduced appetite, Poor hair and skin condition, Pigs may be seen trying to consume urine from other pigs. Over feeding of salt can result in high blood pressure.

Potassium

Function - Works with sodium to assist in correct nerve function and muscular contractions. Assists in maintaining the correct fluid balance in the body. May reduce heart rate.

Source - Green forage, Maize and Molasses.

Herb Sources - Alfalfa, Blue Cohosh, Borage, Carrot leaves,

Chamomile, Coltsfoot, Comfrey, Couch Grass, Centaury, Dandelion, Elder, Eyebright, Fennel, Kelp, Ladies Mantle, Mistletoe, Meadowsweet, Mullein, Nettles, Parsley, Peppermint, Plantain, Raspberry, Shepherds Purse, Skullcap, Wormwood, Yarrow.

Deficiencies - Weight loss, Diarrhea, Muscle weakness.

Zinc

Function - Assists in the metabolism of nutrients. Required for the immune system to function correctly. Needed for healthy skin, hair and hooves. Assists in blood formation.

Sources - Yeast, Bran, Cereal Germ and Zinc Sulphate.

Herb Sources - Kelp and Marshmallow

Deficiencies - Can lead to dry flaky skin, hair loss and poor growth and smaller and fewer piglets. Also could lead to a lowered immune system.

Copper

Function - Essential in the formation of hemoglobin, cartilage and bone. Required for the correct utilization of iron in the body.

Sources - Grassland, Copper, Sulphate, Copper Carbonate.

Herb Sources - Burdock, Chickweed, Chicory, Dandelion, Fennel, Garlic, Horseradish, Kelp, Parsley, Yarrow.

Deficiencies - Brittle weak bones, anemia, faded dull coat, poor iron metabolism, bowing of legs, cardiac and vascular disorders.

Manganese

Function - Required for the utilization of fats and carbohydrates. Essential for the formation of cartilage, assists in the formation of bones and enzymes. Some benefits in pigs can be higher total litter and piglet weight at birth.

Sources - Wheat Bran, Most Grains and Grasslands

Herb Sources - Kelp.

Deficiencies - Deformed piglets whose bones are not correctly developed. Irregular or absent estrous cycles, weak piglets at birth and reduced milk production.

Iron

Function - Essential for the formation of hemoglobin and red blood cells.

Sources - Grasslands and Cereals.

Herb Sources - Alfalfa, Asparagus, Bilberry, Burdock, Blue Cohosh, Cayenne, Chicory, Comfrey, Dandelion, Gentian, Hawthorn, Hops, Mullein, Nettles, Parsley, Raspberry, Skullcap, Vervain, Yellow Dock.

Deficiencies - Anemia, Poor Performance, Poor growth in young stock and maybe labored breathing.

Fluorine

Function - Essential for the formation of healthy teeth and bones, helps prevent tooth decay. Combines with calcium in the body and gives strength to the bones.

Sources - Pasture, Hay, Water and Limestone based supplements.

Herb Sources - Alfalfa, Beet leaves, Garlic, Water Cress.

Deficiencies - Deficiencies are rare but overdosing can occur especially where soils are rich in this mineral and the water has been treated with it as well. Signs of overdosing are discolored, mottled teeth, poor condition and rough coat and lameness in the joints.

Iodine

Function - Needed for correct functioning of the thyroid gland. Required for reproductive cycle to function correctly.

Sources - Kelp, Pasture and Mineral Licks

Herb Sources - Asparagus, Cleavers, Garlic, Kelp, Speedwell, Sarsaparilla.

Deficiencies - Abnormal estrous cycle. Piglets can be still born while others may be hairless and exhibit weakness and deformed joints. Overdosing can lead to enlarged thyroid glands.

Selenium

Function - Works with Vitamin E. Essential part of antioxidant enzymes which help to remove toxins from the system. A component of the amino acids Methionine and Cystine. Assists in maintaining a healthy immune system.

Sources - Pastures, Alfalfa, Fish Meal, Rape Seed meal and Linseed.

Deficiencies - Can be labored breathing and white muscle disease. Overfeeding can cause poisoning. Impaired reproduction, Reduced milk and Mulberry heart disease.

Vitamins

Vitamin A (retinol)

Function - Needed for hormone synthesis, bone growth, and used in most of the mucous membranes of the body. Essential for vision and reproduction.

Sources - Carrots, Carotene in green leafy plants and Cod Liver Oil.

Herb Sources - Alfalfa, Burdock, Cayenne, Comfrey, Dandelion, Kelp, Marshmallow, Papaya, Parsley, Raspberry, Red Clover, Watercress, Yellow Dock.

Deficiencies - Night blindness, Excessive tears, Lack of appetite, Infections of the reproductive tract, Poor growth and weak bones and tendons, in coordination and posterior paralysis.

B1 Thiamine

Function - Assists in metabolizing carbohydrates. Maintains a healthy nervous system. Assists in energy metabolism. This vitamin is made by micro flora in the intestines.

Sources - Good forage, Good hay, Cereal grains Millet, Rice bran and Brewer's Yeast.

Herb Sources - Alfalfa, Burdock, Cayenne, Comfrey, Dandelion, Kelp, Marshmallow, Papaya, Parsley, Raspberry, Red Clover,

Watercress, Yellow Dock.

Deficiencies - Weight loss, Muscular in coordination and missed heart beats. Deficiencies are fairly rare due to this vitamin being made in the intestines.

B2 Riboflavin

Function - Maintains a healthy nervous system. Assists in energy metabolism. This vitamin is also made in the intestines.

Sources - Green forage, Peanut meal, Whey, Brewer's yeast, Good Hay and Milk.

Herb Sources - Alfalfa, Burdock, Fenugreek, Kelp, Parsley, Watercress.

Deficiencies - Rough coat and dry skin, Conjunctivitis, Excessive tearing and may be connected with moon blindness. Hair loss. Deficiencies are fairly rare.

B3 Niacin

Function - Helps in the metabolism of nutrients and also with hormone and lipid syntheses. This vitamin is also made in the intestines.

Sources - Green forage especially Lucerne.

Herb Sources - Alfalfa, Burdock, Fenugreek, Kelp, Parsley, Sage.

Deficiencies - Inflammatory lesions of the GI tract and exhibit diarrhea, weight loss, rough skin and coat and dermatitis on the ears. Over dosing may cause dilation of blood vessels, sickness and itching of skin.

B5 Pantothenic Acid

Function - Assists in energy metabolism and the formation of anti-bodies.

Sources - Green forage, Cereals and Peas.

Deficiencies - Deficiency is rare as this vitamin is made in the intestines.

B6 Pyridoxine

Function - Assists in energy metabolism. maintains health of the nervous system. Assists in the formation of hemoglobin in the blood. Maintains the health of the immune system. May increase litter size. This vitamin is made in the bowel.

Sources - Green forage and Cereal grains.

Herb Sources - Alfalfa, Chlorophyll

Deficiencies - Reduced appetite and growth rate, eye secretions, convulsions, unsteadiness in use of legs.

B12 Cyanocobalamin

Function - Assists in the production of red blood cells. Assists in energy metabolism. Good for stress. Can assist in putting on condition and correcting anemia. Improved reproductive performance. This vitamin is made in the bowel.

Sources - Green forages.

Herb Sources - Alfalfa, Chlorophyll, Dong Quai, Kelp.

Deficiencies - Reduced weight gain, lack of appetite, rough skin and coat, irritability, voice failure and pain and in coordination in the hindquarters.

Biotin

Function - Assists in the metabolism of energy. Maintains sebaceous glands in the skin. Maintains bone marrow. May improve litter number and weight.

Sources - Yeast, Green forage and cereals.

Deficiencies - Excessive hair loss, skin ulceration and dermatitis, eye exudate, inflammation of the mucous membranes of the mouth.

Choline

Function - Assists in the transport of fats stored in the liver to other areas of the body for use as energy. Maintains a healthy nervous system. Structural component of the cell membrane. May increase live pigs born and weaned and improve conception rates.

Sources - Natural Fats, Fish Meal, Green leafy forage, Rapeseed and Yeast cereals.

Deficiencies - Can lead to poor growth and increased storage of fats in the liver. Reduced weight gain, rough hair coat, staggering gate.

Folic Acid

Function - Assists cell metabolism. Required for red blood cell formation. Assists in general metabolism.

Sources - Green leafy forage

Deficiencies - Slow weight gain, fading hair color.

Vitamin C (ascorbic acid)

Function - Essential for the formation of collagen tissue which is vital in tendons and cartilage. Essential for the utilization of essential amino acids lysine and proline. Has a role as a antioxidant. Reported to reduce naval bleeding in new born piglets.

Sources - Made in the liver and other body cells.

Herb Sources - Alfalfa, Burdock, Catnip, Cayenne, Chickweed, Dandelion, Hawthorn, Garlic, Horseradish, Kelp, Parsley, Plantain, Papaya, Raspberry, Rosehips, Shepherds Purse, Yellow Dock.

Deficiencies - None recorded. Supplementation has been given in periods of stress and growth.

Vitamin D

Function - Essential for the absorption of calcium and for growth maintenance and repair of bones and teeth.

Sources - Cut and dried plants, fish oils and through the skin after contact with sunlight.

Herb Sources - Alfalfa, Chlorophyll, Don Quai, Kelp.

Deficiencies - Reduced growth, weak bones and increased bone problems and rickets.

Vitamin E

Function - Helps with the immune system and is a powerful antioxidant. Helps stabilize cell membranes and acts on the reproductive system.

Sources - Leafy green forage, Good hay, Cereals and Alfalfa.

Herb Sources - Alfalfa, Dandelion, Dong Quai, Kelp, Raspberry, rose Hips, Water Cress.

Deficiencies - Anemia, Swelling of joints, muscular in coordination and reduced stamina. Skeletal and cardiac muscle degeneration.

Vitamin K

Function - Helps in the clotting of blood and in calcium assimilation.

Sources - Made in the gut from green leafy forage.

Herb Sources - Alfalfa, Chlorophyll, Plantain, Shepherds Purse.

Deficiencies - Bleeding and longer blood clotting time.

Notes

The Respiratory System

Atrophic Rhinitis

This is a wide spread contagious disease especially in America and Scandinavia and coming to Australia in the early 80s, there are two causative agents.

1/. Bordetella bronchiseptica - associated with the non-progressive form of the disease.

2/. Pasteurella multicoda - associated with the progressive form.

Both types affect the turbinate bones of the nose leading to distortion of the nasal structures. The disease can lead to poor growth among fattening pigs. The severity of the disease is dependent on the virulence of the invading organism and the amount of bacterial toxin absorbed.

Symptoms - Can occur in pigs from 1 to 3 months. In piglets snuffling and sneezing with sometimes difficult breathing are the early signs with the symptoms becoming continuous as the animal grows. Latter a muco-purulent discharge follows. If bleeding from the nostrils occur this is usually one sided. After prolonged sneezing detached portions of the turbinate may be seen in the nasal discharge. Deformity of nasal and facial structures is a constant feature and a twisted snout is a sure pointer to the disease. The upper jaw becomes shortened in relation to the lower while the facial skin develops folds. Sometimes you can pick this pig in a crowd especially at feeding time because the pig will not try to push in to get food and is always trying to protect its snout. It is also disinclined to eat dry food and favors mashes. There is a general retardation of growth.

Herbal Treatment - One of the first herbs to think of here is garlic as garlic is antiviral and antibacterial but the main reason is that garlic exits the body via the mucous membranes hence garlic on your breath when you eat it. The largest mucous membrane in the body are the lungs and also the pipes leading from it. Give Echinacea as well but only for the first month and then stop. Concentrate on the respiratory anti bacterials with a good one being Elecampane. Other herbs to add to a formula would be Eye Bright and Elder. Propolis would be another remedy to consider.

Homoeopathic Treatment

Aurum Metallicum 30C - Used in the treatment of degenerative bone disease affecting the nasal structures, use in the early stage of infection daily for 20 days.

Phosphorus 30C - Hemorrhages accompanying nasal discharge call for this remedy. Also of use in necrotic conditions of the nasal bones. 200C three times daily for 4 weeks.

Silicea 200C - Degeneration of turbinate bones followed by a shedding of tissue. Dose 3 times per week for 3 weeks.

Kali Bichromicum 30C - If discharges are predominantly purulent this remedy should help. Discharges are yellow and stringy. Dose daily for 7 to 10 days.

Pulsatilla 30C - Early signs of sneezing and snuffling in young pigs. Dose daily for 7 days.

Prevention - A nosode could be made from infected material and given on a herd basis.

Cough

While coughing is frequently associated with various pulmonary infections it may arise as a seemingly independent syndrome and takes various forms.

1/. Pleuritic cough - Short and dry and the animal shows pain while coughing.

2/. Bronchitic cough - Starts dry and frequent, becomes moist and soft.

3/. Simple catarrhal cough - Usually moist and infrequent.

4/. Pneumonic Cough - Frequent, may contain rust colored fibrinous deposits in the sputum.

5/. Stomach or intestinal cough - Various forms dependent on alimentary disorders.

Herbal Treatment -Try to figure the cause and decide if you need to build up the immune system with Echinacea and use the antiviral and antibacterial action of Garlic etc. It might be an idea to separate from the herd till you figure it out. Cough is often present in wormy animals long confined in the dusty and vitality impairing atmosphere of stables. I have decided to write the treatment section exactly as it was done in the past and in brackets give you the tinctures used today. For the local relief of the cough give a 1 cup drench of brewed cherry twigs (Wild Cherry Bark Tincture), with one tea spoon of honey and one tea spoon of black treacle added. An alternative and proved excellent drench is a brew of equal parts Pine Needles and Elder twigs, blossoms or leaves (Elder Tincture), 2 handfuls of each of the herbs brewed in a quart of water. Give a drench of one cup. Coltsfoot can replace the Pine or Elder. When mouths are sore or inflamed bathe with a brew of Sage. The following Farrier recipe makes an excellent cough drop which could be used for pigs to - Anise seeds one pound (crush seeds to release the oils) , ground ginger one pound, ground licorice one pound and one handful of caraway seeds. Add sufficient treacle to form a mass and roll into balls. Give slightly less than a half ounce of this mixture every morning and fast the for about a hour allowing it time to work.

Other expectorants to consider are Fenugreek, Hyssop, Horehound, Mullein and Thyme. If the cough is harsh and painful sounding consider these **Demulcent Herbs** - Coltsfoot, Comfrey, Fenugreek, Licorice, Marshmallow, Mullein and Plantain.

Homoeopathic Treatment

Bryonia 6C - Pleuritic cough, dry, symptoms worse on movement, better from pressure or pressure over the affected area. Dose 3 times daily for 3 days.

Belladonna 30C - Cough accompanied by full pulse, dry cough, hot smooth skin, dilated pupils, nervous symptoms. Dose every 2 hours for 4 doses.

Drosera 6C - Spasmodic coughs of a chronic nature, sometimes associated with asthmatic symptoms worse at night when the animal lies down. Dose every 2 hours for 4 doses.

Nux Vom 6C - Origin in digestive upsets, dry cough, hoarse, spasmodic worse in the morning. Dose 3 times daily for 3 days.

Causticum 30C - Cough relieved by drinking, expectorations scanty. Dose night and morning for 4 days.

Arsenic Alb 1M - Cough worse after midnight, animal restless, thirsty with dry skin, cough worse after drinking even small quantities. Dose night and morning for 4 days.

Spongia 30C - Cough worse on inspiration and worse towards midnight, relieved by drinking, sometimes associated with heart disease. Dose night and morning for 3 days.

Sticta 6C - Cough originates more in trachea, is worse in the evening and during the night and on inspiration. Dose 3 times daily for 3 days.

Swine Influenza - Hog Flu

A acute infectious disease caused by the porcine virus strain Influenza A to which pigs are the main host with the infection being spread through the air. Has a sudden onset and mainly effects the respiratory tract, recovery can be expected except in those cases where it turns into pneumonia. Variations in weather temperature can trigger an outbreak and most animals in the herd are liable to get it. Mortality is low except in young piglets. Can cause abortions and maybe weak litters.

Symptoms - Most animals in the herd are likely to have this or are about to get it. Onset is sudden with loss of appetite a early sign, fever to 108F or 42C, similarly effected animals may huddle together and there is a disinclination to move, breathing become labored and is through an open mouth. Progression to pneumonia is indicated by the severity of the respiratory symptoms including abdominal breathing. If animals are made to move this brings on coughing which is harsh and dry. The temperature remains high while outward signs may include conjunctivitis and nasal discharge. In uncomplicated infections the course of the disease is usually 3 to 7 days with the recovery usually as fast as the onset.

Herbal Treatment

One of the first herbs to think of here is garlic as garlic is antiviral and antibacterial but the main reason is that garlic exits the body via the mucous membranes hence garlic on your breath when you eat it. Give Echinacea as well but only for the first month and then stop. Give high doses of vitamin C. The main herbs used for flu like symptoms are Elder, Golden Rod, Eye Bright and Catmint. For the fever think of the Diaphoretic herbs like Yarrow, Peppermint, Penny Royal, Angelica.

Homoeopathic Treatment

Aconitum 10M - The first remedy to use as soon as the symptoms appear especially in the others in the herd as it may stop the disease from happening if you're lucky. Use one dose every hour for 4 doses.

Gelsemium 200C - Listlessness and prostration indicate this remedy which has traditionally been used for bad doses of the flu. Use one dose every hour for 3 doses followed by one 3 times daily for 2 days.

Bryonia 30C - Disinclination to move is the keynote of this remedy. Any movement brings on coughing and distress. Use one dose 3 times daily for 5 days

Phosphorus 200C - Severe cases with pneumonia complications with breathing out of the mouth and a harsh dry cough. Use one dose twice daily for 2 days followed by a 1M dose daily for 4 days.

Dulcamara 200C - If the onset was the result of exposure to cold nights after warm days or from exposure to damp think of this remedy. Use twice daily for 5 days.

Bronchitis

Inflammation of the bronchial mucous membranes may arise independently of other illnesses or may be a sequel to another problem or catarrhal state. It may arise simply by exposure to cold dry winds or to damp and cold or may be due to some foreign body irritating the mucous membranes usually as a result of dusty and powdery feeds or from poor drenching. Try to remove all causes.

Symptoms - Loss of appetite, elevation of temperature, pulse becomes full and quick accompanied by a frequent pain full cough but is paroxysmal and incomplete. The inspiration is incomplete short and painful and the expiration is prolonged. Mucous secretion soon becomes purulent and may run from the nose as well as appear in the cough. Rattling respiratory sounds can be herd over the rib area.

Herbal Treatment

The treatment is fairly much the same as Colds and Coughs. Here are a list of some other Herbs that are very good for the treatment of bronchitis with most of them being expectorants - Elecampane (anti-bacterial action as well), Coltsfoot, Grindelia, Mullein, Pleurisy Root, Horehound and Comfrey

Demulcent Herbs - Coltsfoot, Comfrey, Fenugreek, Licorice, Marshmallow, Mullein and Plantain.

For cases that seem to be lasting a long time think of giving Fenugreek which over time thins the mucous out and stimulates the lymphatic system to start cleaning the area out.

Homoeopathic Treatment

Aconite 6C - Early stages, with hot dry skin, feverish symptoms and anxious expression. Dose hourly for 4 doses

Belladonna 1M - Pulse full and bounding, with dilated pupils, sweating and excitement. Dose every 2 hours for 4 doses.

Ant Tart 30C - Moist cough with threatened pulmonary edema, Rattling sounds may be heard in the chest, respirations increased. Dose 3 times daily for 3 days.

Bryonia 6C - Cough hard and dry, pleura becomes affected, relief from pressure over the ribs. Dose 3 time daily for 3 days.

Dulcamara 6C - Condition has origins from damp surroundings and coughing worse after exertion. Dose 3 times daily for 3 days.

Kali Bich 200C - Phlegm in bronchial tubes difficult to expel, nasal discharge. Dose 3 times daily for 3 days.

Drosera 6C - Coughing becomes spasmodic in character, paroxysms follow one another rapidly. Dose 3 times daily for 4 days.

Spongia 6C - Bouts of coughing eased by eating or drinking, worse by exposure to cold air. Dose 3 times daily for 4 days.

Enzootic Pneumonia

Found in most countries and is a bacterial like organism known as Mycoplasma hypopneumonia which causes an infection that spreads easily through the herd and opens the way for secondary infections. The disease is a low grade long term Pneumonia. Both growth rate and feed conversion are badly affected. This disease is wide spread in Australia. The death rate is low. There is an incubation period of 10 to 16 days and the bacteria are rapidly inactivated by disinfectants used to clean the living quarters. Pigs of all ages are susceptible and the old and mature pigs may never really fully recover.

Symptoms - Coughing develops which soon becomes chronic and may last for many months. The intensity of the coughing is worse in growing and fattening pigs. There is a loss of appetite and a rise in temperature at the acute stage, breathing has been described as labored or thumping, severely infected pigs become prostrate and are disinclined to move.

Herbal Treatment

One of the first herbs to think of here is garlic as garlic is antiviral and antibacterial but the main reason is that garlic exits the body via the mucous membranes hence garlic on your breath when you eat it. Give Echinacea as well but only for the first month and then stop. Give high doses of vitamin C. Look at the section on Cough and Flu to get the remedies for coughing and fever. Herbs to consider are Pleurisy Root, Mullein, Fenugreek, Elder and Angelica. Upon recovery keep up the Fenugreek as this is a rubbish remover and a multi vitamin pill in one and add to it carrots which are high in vitamin A as we want this to help reduce the scaring in the lungs.

Homoeopathic Treatment

See Cough for extra remedies.

Aconitum 10M - The first remedy to use as soon as the symptoms appear especially in the others in the herd as it may stop the disease from happening if you're lucky. Use one dose every hour for 4 doses.

Phosphorus 10M - Important remedy when pneumonia is well established. Breathing is labored and the cough is rough and dry. Give a dose 3 times daily for 3 days.

Bryonia 30C - Disinclination to move is the keynote of this remedy. Any movement brings on coughing and distress. Use one dose 3 times daily for 5 days

Mycoplasma Nosode 30C - Use on a daily basis for 10 days together with the appropriate remedy.

Prevention - M. Hyopneumonia 30C should be employed on a herd basis.

Haemophilus Pleuropneumonia

This disease is widely distributed and is a severe rapidly developing disease causing a large number of deaths (25% to 50%) in affected herds with survivors having reduced growth rates and a persistent cough. Onset is sudden and spread is rapid, Infection spreads throughout the body and in severe cases there is bleeding in to the lung tissues and excess fluid in the chest. Survivors become carriers. Pigs of all ages are susceptible though it is primarily a disease of growing pigs. The spread of the infection is airborne by droplets. Incubation may be from 3 days to 3 weeks.

Symptoms - In the animals that suddenly die the symptoms can be temperature rise, vomiting, diarrhea with little or no respiratory symptoms except for breathing difficulty breathing before death along with frothy blood stained mucous from the mouth and nostrils. In the acute form there is a rise in temperature up to 107F or 41.5C, loss of appetite followed by a appearance of depression together with coughing and difficulty in breathing. Cyanosis due to involvement of the heart may take place. The chronic form may follow the acute stage where the temperature remains normal, loss of appetite, there may be coughing and arthritis or in some outbreaks there are chronic abscesses in different parts of the body.

Herbal Treatment

Treatment is the same as above but isolate the animal or quarantine the effected animals. One of the first herbs to think of here is garlic as garlic is antiviral and antibacterial but the main reason is that garlic exits the body via the mucous membranes hence garlic on your breath when you eat it. Give Echinacea as well but only for the first month and then stop. Give high doses of vitamin C.. Look at the section on Cough and Flu to get the remedies for coughing and fever. Herbs to consider are Pleurisy Root, Mullein, Fenugreek, Elder and Angelica.   In cases like this where death is a possibility think of using Astragalus not only for its immune enhancing actions but because it helps the body work with less oxygen. Upon recovery keep up the Fenugreek as this is a rubbish remover and a multi vitamin pill in one and add to it carrots which are high in vitamin A as we want this to help reduce the scaring in the lungs.

Homoeopathic Treatment

Aconitum 10M - The first remedy to use as soon as the symptoms appear especially in the others in the herd as it may stop the disease from happening if you're lucky. Use one dose every hour for 4 doses.

Arsenicum Album 1M- Diarrhea and vomiting could be contained by the use of this remedy. Use daily for 5 days.

Echinacea 3C - Septicemia involvement in young pigs may be controlled with this remedy. Use three times daily for 7 days.

Phosphorus 30C - Beneficial in controlling respiratory symptoms associated with acute cases. Use twice daily for 5 days.

Acidum Salicylicum 200C - If arthritis develops this may prove useful. Dose3 times per week for 4 weeks

Silicea 30C - This is used for the abscesses if they appear. Dose daily for 7 days.

Preventation - A nosode could be made from infected material and given on a herd basis.

Pleurisy

Pleurisy is an inflammation of the serous membranes lining the chest cavity and enveloping the lungs. Injuries to the chest may lead to pleurisy and it may also arise from exposure to cold and damp though is seldom seen as a sole condition in Pigs. Acute Pleurisy is usually secondary to Pneumonia or Pericarditis.

Symptoms - Acute form is of sudden onset accompanied by lack of appetite, a rise in temperature and evidence of Pneumonia over the chest wall. In the first stage there is great pain aggravated by movement and the animal may be stiff and still, the pulse is quick and hard with the breathing abdominal and the chest being fixed as far as possible with the inspiration short and jerky and the expiration longer. The pain is caused by the friction of the dry inflamed pleural surfaces of the lung and chest rubbing against each other. At this stage the ear detects a dry friction murmur resembling somewhat the sound made by rubbing to pieces of sole leather together. Pressure between the ribs gives pain and usually causes the animal to grunt. The muzzle is hot and dry. Respirations are increased when secondary to Pneumonia. From here the disease will either get better or worse and in unfavorable cases death occurs during the second or third week from asphyxia or heart failure.

Herbal Treatment

Start the treatment the same as Pneumonia and refer to the other respiratory conditions for treatment for the different symptoms.

Below is a summary of how a herbalist would approach the condition using herbal tinctures. If you can get hold of the herbs mentioned below you could make a very effective formula for helping this condition. Read up on each mentioned herb.

Pleurisy is an infection so we shall attack the infection directly with Echinacea and Garlic, fever can also be a large part of pleurisy so we well attack this symptom with the herbs that are called diaphoretics which are herbs used for fevers, some of them are Yarrow, Peppermint and Ginger. As there is a lot of pain with this condition we shall add some demulcent (soothing Herbs) herbs which will hopefully sooth the effected membranes and reduce the pain, a good one here to use is Mullein and I would also be inclined to add Elecampane and Comfrey for its all-round effect. For the Anti-Inflammatory herbs it would be a toss-up between Angelica and Golden Rod as these are both good all round herbs and their actions cover most of the symptoms of this disease. So a possible good formula we could make would be Echinacea, Garlic, Mullein, Yarrow and Angelica at about 20% each so it is easy to make up. Try to make your formulas no more than five herbs at a time and try to base them on the actions you need. If this was a serious case I would also add Astragalus for the reasons mentioned under Pneumonia.

And of course we can't forget to mention Pleurisy Root.

Homoeopathic Treatment

Aconite 6C - The early febrile stage. Dose hourly for 4 doses.

Arsenicum 30C - Chronic pleurisy may be relieved by this remedy, useful for cases that are slow to respond. Dose 2 times daily for 7 days.

Belladonna 1M - Pulse full and bounding, with dilated pupils, sweating and excitement. Dose every 2 hours for 4 doses.

Bryonia 30C - Better at rest, pressure over pleural area relieves, cough usually hard and dry, resents movement prefers to lie down, Dose every 2 hours for 4 doses.

Apis 30C - Edema occurs in pleural cavities, there may be accompanying brisket edema, urine scanty and high colored. Dose 3 times daily for 3 days

Cantharis 200C - Pleural effusion, mucous expectorated with cough is usually blood stained, severe straining when trying to pass urine.

Kali Carb 200C - Symptoms of pain worse on right side, cough worse in early morning and there is usually a dry throat. Dose 3 times daily for 3 days.

Phosphorus 200C - A main remedy once hepatisation has set in, pressure resented particularly on the left side, sputum is rust colored, trembling of the body, follows well after Aconite or Bryonia.

Sulphur 6C - Use in the convalescent stage of pleurisy. Dose once daily for 6 days.

Herbal Overview of The Respiratory System

Always start off with Echinacea and Garlic as you never know how violent the condition will become as this can save problems later, also consider fasting the animal. Below are the Actions to think of when dealing with the Respiratory System. As usual isolate the animal and observe. Consider also if the condition is affecting another system? Is there diarrhea, is there any unusual behavior, is there fever, what is the temperature, is the animal anxious etc. Some of the best herbs for this system are Angelica, Coltsfoot, Comfrey, Elder, Elecampane, Eyebright, Fenugreek, Golden Rod, Hyssop, Horehound, Horse Radish, Licorice, Mullein, Myrrh, Plantain, Sage and Thyme.

Anti-biotic - Chaparral, Echinacea, Elecampane, Garlic, Myrrh.

Anti-catarrhal - Helps the body to remove excess catarrhal build ups.

Herbs - Cayenne, Coltsfoot, Cranesbill, Echinacea, Elder, Eyebright, Garlic, Golden Rod, Hyssop, Marshmallow, Mullein, Myrrh, Peppermint, Sage, Thyme, Yarrow.

Anti-inflammatory - Helps the body to combat inflammations. Herbs mentioned under demulcents will often act in this way especially when they coat sore throats and pipe lines.

Herbs - Angelica, Comfrey, Cranesbill, Eyebright, Feverfew, Ginger, Golden Rod, Lady's Mantle, Licorice, Marshmallow.

Anti-microbial - Helps the body destroy or resist pathogenic micro-organisms.

Herbs - Aniseed, Echinacea, Garlic, Myrrh, Peppermint, Plantain,

Rosemary, Sage, Thyme.

Antispasmodic - Prevents or eases spasms and cramps.

Herbs - Aniseed, Angelica, Coltsfoot, Fennel, Horehound, Hyssop, Mullein, Rosemary, Sage, Skullcap, Thyme

Anti-viral - Astragalus, Echinacea, Garlic, Myrrh?, Shitake, St John's Wort, Pau D'Arco.

Anthelmintic - Destroys or expels worms from the digestive system.

Herbs - Garlic, Tansy, Wormwood, Thyme, Rue.

Astringent - Contracts tissue which in turn reduces discharges, these herbs contain tannins.

Herbs - Agrimony, Angelica, Comfrey, Elecampane, Eyebright, Golden Rod, Marshmallow, Mullein, Myrrh, Plantain, Sage, Rosemary, Shepherds Purse, Thyme.

Demulcent - Soothes and protects irritated or inflamed internal tissues.

Herbs - Coltsfoot, Comfrey, Fenugreek, Licorice, Marshmallow, Mullein, Oats, Plantain.

Diaphoretic - Aids the skin in the elimination of toxins and produces sweat thus reducing the temperature of fevers.

Herbs - Angelica, Cayenne, Elder, Elecampane, Fennel, Garlic, Ginger, Golden Rod, Hyssop, Peppermint, Thyme, Yarrow.

Expectorant - Supports the body in the removal of excess mucous from the respiratory system and helps in the control of coughs.

Herbs -Angelica, Aniseed, Coltsfoot, Comfrey, Elder, Elecampane, Fennel, Fenugreek, Garlic, Hyssop, Horehound, Licorice, Marshmallow, Mullein, Myrrh, Plantain, Sweet Violets, Thyme.

Febrifuge - Helps the body to bring down fevers.

Herbs - Cayenne, Elder Flowers, Hyssop, Marigold, Penny Royal, Peppermint, Plantain, Raspberry, Sage, Thyme, Vervain.

Immune Booster - Astragalus, Echinacea, Reshi, Shitake.

Pectoral - Has a general strengthening and healing effect on the respiratory system.

Herbs - Aniseed, Coltsfoot, Comfrey, Elder, Garlic, Hyssop, Licorice, Mullein, Horehound.

Notes

The Digestive System

Enteric Colibacillosis

This is a common disease in nursing and weaning pigs. E. Coli is a normal inhabitant of gut flora where its function is to break down food particles and render them suitable for absorption. Disease is likely to occur when under stress, weather changes, prolonged exposure to damp conditions or deprivation of colostrum in the young pig. The toxins of this bacteria cause fluids and electrolytes to be secreted into the intestinal lumen which results in diarrhea, dehydration and acidosis. This particular condition is associated with diarrhea in pigs from 3 days old to post weaning. Hemorrhagic gastroenteritis develops in older pigs.

Symptoms - Diarrhea varies to the virulence of the invading organism. Dehydration follows. Outbreaks may affect whole litters or single pigs. Faeces vary from whitish or creamy to light brown. Vomiting occurs in some of the animals accompanied by loss of bodyweight. The muscles of the abdomen become flaccid, the skin may be bluish or gray extending to around the anal area, Diarrhea is less severe in older pigs. Gastroenteritis with bloody stools is confined to older weaned pigs. Cyanosis of the extremities sometimes develops in these cases.

Herbal Treatment

Start with a strong purge of castor oil so as to try to get as much of the toxin making bacteria out of the body as fast as you can. Next think of the astringent herbs as these close the pores and may stop or slow down the fluids that are being secreted in the lumen, try the strong ones such as Cranesbill and Shepherds purse. All strong astringents also have an antibacterial action which we really need in this case. Fast the animal but keep it near water and also start dosing with Garlic and Echinacea. Latter think of Slippery Elm for its astringent but soothing demulcent action and also for its nutritional value. See diarrhea and Scours.

Homoeopathic Treatment

Coli-Gaertner 30C - The combined nosodes of E coli and Gaertner have been given with good results. Give one dose daily for 7 days.

China 6C - Dehydration and weakness associated with fluid loss will be helped by this remedy. Give one dose 3 times daily for 4 days.

Arsenicum 1M - Light brown diarrhea with or without vomiting indicates this remedy. Give twice daily for 5 days.

Lachesis 30C - Purplish or dark blue lesions on the skin indicate this remedy especially if they occur over the lower flank. Give three times daily for 7 days.

Diarrhea and Dysentery (Enteritis)

Diarrhea is purging or looseness of the bowels in which the discharges are faecal. Causes can be improper food, putrid water, worms, Cobalt and Copper deficiencies, exposure to damp and cold weather and as a result of a debilitated constitution. The best cure is by removing the cause. Dysentery can follow neglected diarrhea.

Symptoms - Dung is loose latter becomes liquid and is sometimes spurted out to a distance, there may or may not be griping pains. If the animal retains strength and appetite the diarrhea may be regarded as a effort of nature to remove some unhealthy matter and should not be stopped. Long continued and violent diarrhea must be treated.

Herbal Treatment

The best cure here is to try and remove the cause and if the condition gets worse treat as dysentery. If the problem looks serious give a laxative drench to sweep the putrid matter from the intestines. A quick effective drench is one or two ounces of Epsom Salts dissolved in a pint brew of Dill Seed water (one small handful of dill seeds boiled for 5 minutes). Senna Pods can also be used as a laxative drench. Fast the animal for 24 hours following the drench and give a garlic brew or tablets in the evening for internal disinfecting. Reintroduce food slowly, but add to this Slippery Elm which will soothe and gently astringe the intestines along with adding nourishment.

Dysentery is inflammation of the mucous membranes of the bowels attended with increased secretion of mucous, pain, sometimes blood and with increased straining. This can also be part and a symptom of a more serious disease such as enterotoxaemia, Coccidiosis or some plant poisoning such as Deadly Nightshade.

Symptoms - There may be loss of spirits and appetite, slight gripping pains and frequent straining passing a quantity of wind and mucous usually mixed with blood or with shreds of mucous membrane and there may be fever.

Herbal Treatment

Treatment is similar to Diarrhea. If case is severe start off with a laxative drench maybe something a bit stronger such as Castor Oil. Cease all food for at least 24 hours maybe more. Slippery Elm is our main herb for Dysentery as it is mildly astringent and very demulcent and in this case mix it with lots of honey so as to encourage eating as well as making it very nutritious. To this we add about 10 garlic capsules which are there to disinfect the bowel along with some chlorophyll and a hand full of charcoal with these last 2 being there to cleanse and absorb the toxins and gas. As the intestines heal milk should be added to the Slippery Elm and honey gruel along with 1 small teaspoon full of Gentian to one and a half pints of gruel

Homoeopathic Treatment

Aconite 30C - Diarrhea in the primary stage, at the beginning of acute cases that come on suddenly and violently, when it arises from taking cold, considerable fever, inflammation of the bowels, can be alternated with Nux Vom. Dose every half hour for 4 doses.

Nux Vom 12X - Discharges slimy and offensive with rumbling noises in the bowels and passing of wind, when there are symptoms of indigestion and when purging is alternated with constipation. Dose once every 2 hours.

Arsenicum 1M - For watery, slimy, greenish or brownish diarrhea, with or without gripping pains and can smell offensive, great rumbling in the bowels and flatulence, total loss of appetite and a marked prostration of strength, skin and extremities cold great restlessness. Dose every hour for 4 doses.

China 30C - Useful in chronic cases or when caused by hot weather and not of a inflammatory character, painless discharge, loss of appetite and strength. Can be used as a tonic when acute symptoms have passed away, evacuations consist partly of undigested food , can be pain during discharge.

Bryonia 30C- If the disorder has been brought on by a change of temperature especially from hot to cold, by drinking cold water or impure water, faeces are very watery and involuntary passed and may contain undigested food, can be alternating diarrhea and constipation. Dose four times a day.

Mercurius Cor 200C- Frequent discharge of mucous tinged with blood or thin bloody and fetid stools, frequent urging to stool, redness and swollen appearance of the anus, symptoms worse at night. Dose 3 times daily for 3 days.

Colocynthis 6C - Nausea, severe colicky pains, slimy evacuations or mucous tinged with blood, distension of the bowels and pain on pressure, tenesmus, thirst, variable temperature of the body being at one time shivering and soon after very hot. Dose every half hour for 4 doses.

Chamomilla 30C- If there is pain just before a evacuation which can be of a greenish colour with mucous. Dose four times a day

Scour (Indigestion and Dysentery in Piglets)

Causes may be similar to indigestion. Pathogenic strains of E coli are the most common causes of scour in sucking and weaned pigs. Other causes may be a acid and alkali imbalance, failure to ingest colostrum after birth, lack of sanitation or worms and in this case it would be worthwhile finding out the names of the worms so you can treat all the stock

Symptoms - The piglet is depressed, the appetite is poor, sometimes there is fever, the extremities may be cold along with the nose and there may be a rapid and weak pulse. The dung becomes gradually softer and lighter in color until it is cream colored and a little thicker then milk. It has a most offensive odor and may contain clumps of curd. There may be pain on passing dung and also abdominal colicky pains. In severe cases there is sudden prostration with great weakness and without treatment will lead to death. A frequent sequel can be Pneumonia.

With Piglets there can be 3 stages that the scour may come in.

1/. The first stage may occur a few days after birth or after the 36 hours which is when the antibody level in the colostrum declines. Consider changing the environment if possible so they can get away from the causing bacteria.

2/. The 2nd peak time is at 2 to 3 weeks of age and is often referred to as milk scours and is usually less severe than the first. At this stage E coli is well established in the gut and the piglets may be eating small amounts of food. Remember a clean living area is most important for the young. Stress is another factor to consider.

3/. Weaning Time especially in pigs weaned between 14 and 28 days of age. In the piglet of this age the passive immunity of the colostrum has worn off and the immune system is still immature. Another hazard is that bacteria can multiply in undigested food and the digestive system is not mature enough as well. Consider also stress for this is also a major change of life for the piglet.

Herbal Treatment

Remove the cause, give the appropriate feed of best quality in small doses. If being bottle fed make sure all utensils are clean. The speediest cure for very young scouring bottle fed piglets is to let them suck from a healthy mother. For older piglets treatment should begin with a laxative drench to sweep the putrid matter out of the intestines. A quick effective drench is 1 or 2 ounces of Epsom's salts dissolved in 1 and a half pints of a brew of Dill seed and water or Senna pods. (One hand full of Dill seeds brewed for 15 minutes in 1 and half pints of water.) After this fast the young piglet making sure they are warm and comfortable for 24 hours and give some garlic capsules in the evening for internal disinfecting. On the second day give 3 meals of milk mixed with the same amount of water, add to this 1 teaspoon full of molasses and then the main ingredient which is slippery elm. If the piglet is not eating give some of this in a drench and see what happens. Make sure there is lots of fresh clean water especially if it is a hot day as the young dehydrates fairly fast. Towards the end of the third day slowly introduce its normal food but very carefully.

Homoeopathic Treatment

Look at the remedies listed under Diarrhea and Dysentery especially China in long standing cases, other remedies are listed below.

Aconite 30C - Diarrhea in the primary stage, at the beginning of acute cases that come on suddenly and violently, when it arises from taking cold, considerable fever, inflammation of the bowels, can be alternated with Nux Vom. Dose every half hour for 4 doses.

Cuprum Aceticum 6C - A useful remedy for scouring, the abdomen is usually tympanic prior to evacuation, stools may be dark with blood stained mucous, animal is generally weak and trembling. Dose every 2 hours for 4 doses followed by one twice daily for 3 days.

Veratrum Album 30C - General appearance of collapse with signs of abdominal pain preceding the onset of diarrhea, stools are watery and forcibly evacuated, body sweating is present, the pig is cold and there may be a bluish tinge to the mucous membranes. Dose every 2 hours for 4 doses.

Carbo Veg 200C - Stools are preceded by signs of abdominal colic with flatulence, it is a excellent remedy for helping revive apparently moribund patients, such pigs should be given access to fresh air. Dose every hour for 4 doses.

Dulcamara 30C - A useful remedy if the onset of disease symptoms is associated with exposure to damp, Dose 3 times daily for 2 days.

Mercurius Cor 200C- Frequent discharge of mucous tinged with blood or thin bloody and fetid stools, frequent urging to stool, redness and swollen appearance of the anus, symptoms worse at night. Dose 3 times daily for 3 days.

Note - Emergency Rehydration Liquid (electrolytes)

Homemade Electrolyte Solution

Since death results from dehydration and shock the first goal is to restore the electrolyte balance.

2 tablespoons of salt

1 teaspoon of baking soda

8 tablespoons of honey

1 gallon of water.

Swine Dysentery

Also known as Vibrionic Dysentery. This is a severe muco-heamorrhagic disease affecting the large intestines. Mainly infects growing pigs over 8 weeks old. The cause is from a spirochaetal called Serpulino hyodysenteriae which proliferates in the large intestines causing degeneration and inflammation of the superficial mucosa causing bleeding in some places and hyper secretion of mucous. The organism does not penetrate beyond the intestines. The disease can be severe with a high death rate or run a milder course resulting in poor growth rates. Whip worm infection in pigs exacerbates the effects of swine dysentery. The disease is worldwide. Always quarantine new pigs.

Symptoms - There is diarrhea in all cases but the severity varies due to the virulence of the infection. There might be a slight rise in temperature along with partial anorexia. At first the stools are soft and of a yellow gray color then after a few days become mucous and blood stained. The back becomes arched and there are signs of abdominal pain. Thirst and dehydration along with emaciation result in well-established infections. Chronic infections show dark blood stained scouring with the pig being very dehydrated, weak, gaunt and emaciated.

Herbal Treatment

If you know it is this disease start with a strong purge of castor oil so as to try to get as much of the toxin making bacteria out of the body as fast as you can. We need to try to stop this disease at the beginning as in all similar problems before the damage is done. Next think of the astringent herbs as these close the pores and may stop or slow down the fluids that are being secreted in the lumen, try the strong ones such as Cranesbill and Shepherds purse. All strong astringents also have a antibacterial action which we really need in this case. Fast the animal but keep it near water and also start dosing with Garlic and Echinacea. Latter think of Slippery Elm for its astringent but soothing demulcent action and also for its nutritional value. Isolate the pig from the others especially after the purge has taken effect. See diarrhea and Scours.

Homoeopathic Treatment

Aconitum 10M - If the early temperature rise is noted in time this remedy will help. Dose every hour for 4 doses.

Iris Versicolor 30C - Early soft stool call for this remedy. There is usually tenderness over the area of the liver. Dose 3 times daily for 7 days.

Colocynthis 1M - Arching of the back with abdominal pain are the leading symptoms for this remedy. Dose twice daily for 5 days.

Phosphorus 30C - Animals with thirst and early blood flecked stools may be helped by this remedy. Vomiting is occasionally present. Dose 3 times daily for 5 days.

Arsenicum Album 1M - This remedy matches the more chronic form of the disease. Dose daily for 10 days.

Porcine Rotavirus

Viruses of this group are associated with gastro enteritis and diarrhea and are a common disease with pigs of all ages being susceptible but suckers and post wearers being affected the most. Young piglets deprived of colostrum are very susceptible to this disease. The virus is ingested and then attacks the small intestines damaging the walls causing malabsorption and osmotic diarrhea.

Symptoms - There is a incubation period of 12 to 24 hours after which loss of appetite sets in accompanied by intermittent vomiting, profuse yellowish white diarrhea follows leading to dehydration. Older pigs are less likely to be affected by dehydration and diarrhea. The majority of adult animals are immune to these viruses but infection is common in the younger age groups. Diarrhea often begins in pigs 5 days to 3 weeks old, or immediately after weaning (not getting anti-bodies from milk). The feces of nursing pigs often are yellow or gray and pasty in their early stages and progress to gray and pasty after 2 days. Diarrhea persists for up to 2 to 5 days. Diarrheic pigs become gaunt and rough haired but mortality is usually low. Weaned pigs have watery feces that contain poorly digested feed and can become lethargic with emaciation.

Herbal Treatment

Start treatment as mentioned in Enteric Colibacillosis. Dose with Garlic and Echinacea so as to attack virus and raise immunity. Astragalus is another good anti-viral to think of. Licorice is a good herb to think of for its anti-inflammatory action and especially for its demulcent and soothing action as this will be needed on the inside of the small intestine. Peppermint and Aniseed could be used together for their pain killing and carminative actions as well as all their other actions. We need a strong astringent to stop fluid leaking into the intestines so think of Cranesbill and Shepherds Purse as these are the strongest. These herbs may be combined and dosed together. Isolate and observe.

Homoeopathic Treatment

Arsenic Album 1M - Should be considered to control early vomiting and may also stop the progression to enteritis and diarrhea. Dose every hour for 4 doses.

Veratrum Alb 30C - Excellent remedy in helping to control diarrhea, the stools have a rice water like appearance. Dose 3 times daily for 7 days.

Camphora 30C - Dehydration due to excess loss of fluid should be helped by this remedy. Symptoms may come on suddenly and progress rapidly. Dose every hour for 4 doses followed by 3 times daily for 3 days.

China Off 6C - Useful to control dehydration but symptoms are less severe than in the previous remedy. Dose 3 times daily for 7 days.

Phosphorus 200C - If vomiting is the more prominent symptom use this remedy. Dose 3 times daily for 5 days.

Rotavirus Nosode 30C - Combine with any selected remedy . Dose daily for 5 days.

Transmissible Gastroenteritis

Referred to as TGE. This is a highly contagious disease that causes vomiting and diarrhea in pigs of all ages but affects piglets under 2 weeks of age the worst. The virus is associated with the Coronavirus group and out breaks are more often seen in the winter months as the virus survives better in the cold. The infection spread rapidly by the air or contact exposure. The virus attacks the small intestine in the areas of the jejunum and ileum damaging the mucosa and causing malabsorption, diarrhea and dehydration. The death rate is usually high in a outbreak. With piglets over a month old having a better chance of survival. Older animals can become infected but rarely suffer from severe complications. Farrowing time is the greatest risk time for infection being passed on to the suckers.

Symptoms - Has a incubation period of 18 hours to 3 days. Vomiting is the initial sign. There may be occasional vomiting followed by a watery yellowish diarrhea. Affected animals soon lose weight and dehydration develops, with the animal showing a excessive thirst. Rapid spread of the condition leads to a high mortality rate. Diarrhea is profuse and faeces may contain undigested milk. The death rate is nearly 100% in pigs less the 1 week old while pigs over a year seldom die. For the older age groups there may be diarrhea which is usually mild together with loss of appetite, lactating sows may experience a loss of milk.

Herbal Treatment

Treat as written up under Rotavirus.

Homoeopathic Treatment

Aconite 30C- Diarrhea in the primary stage, at the beginning of acute cases that come on suddenly and violently, when it arises from taking cold, considerable fever, inflammation of the bowels, can be alternated with Nux Vom. Dose every half hour for 4 doses.

Veratrum Alb 30C - Excellent remedy in helping to control diarrhea, the stools have a rice water like appearance. Dose 3 times daily for 7 days.

Camphora 30C - Dehydration due to excess loss of fluid should be helped by this remedy. Symptoms may come on suddenly and progress rapidly. Dose every hour for 4 doses followed by 3 times daily for 3 days.

China 30C - Useful in chronic cases and not of a inflammatory character, painless discharge, loss of appetite and strength. Can be used as a tonic when acute symptoms have passed away, evacuations consist partly of undigested food , can be pain during discharge.

NOTE - As the danger time is more at farrowing time consider giving a Nosode at 30C of the disease to sows during the last month of their pregnancy. Dose 3 times per week and then give the Nosode to each piglet at birth.

Salmonellosis

There are 2 main organisms S cholerae and S typhinurium with the latter being the worst. Weaned pigs are the main group to suffer from this infection. Recovered animals remain carriers. Sources of infection include carrier pigs, rodents, contaminated feed and premises. Try to keep the rat and mice population to a minimum. Stress can make the animals more susceptible to this disease. Infected pigs when slaughtered becomes a source of infection for humans handling and eating the contaminated carcass. Treatment of Antibiotics given to the animal are of no benefit.

Symptoms - Infection by these bacteria can cause a wide variety of conditions and symptoms ranging from septicemia, colitis to pneumonia. Less commonly meningitis, encephalitis and abortion are encountered. Weaned pigs less than 5 months old are susceptible to the septiceamic form less commonly are the older pigs effected. The pigs shows a disinclination to move and the appetite is lost. Temperature may rise to 107 F, a moist cough develops and a purple discoloration is seen on the extremities. Yellow faeces show after about 4 days and the death rate is high.

The enterocolic form is seen in pigs from weaning till 4 months of age with acute and chronic forms recognized as probably S typhinurium. The Faeces are watery and yellow and the diarrhea may last up to 7 days. Relapses are common in the more chronic form with the occasional blood stained stools.

Herbal Treatment

Isolate the animal immediately from the others and provide fluid with electrolytes and a clean warm dry environment. You have to decide here whether it is worth treating the animal or destroying it, if I had young kids I would destroy it. Treat as written up under Rotavirus but consider the following increase the dose of Echinacea as this is the main herb for septicemia and think about adding Sarsaparilla and Burdock to the mix of herbs as these are both blood cleansers. Treat the symptoms as you see them happening. For the fever look under the action Diaphoretic and try to find a herb that can give you many useful actions such as Peppermint, Fennel and Ginger.

Homoeopathic Treatment

Aconitum 10M - Use for acute infections coming on suddenly. One dose every hour for 4 doses.

Pyrogen 1M - A good remedy for septicemia especially if the pulse doesn't match the temperature. Dose 3 times daily for 2 days.

Lachesis 30C - Purplish discoloration of the extremities and the abdomen call for this remedy. Dose 3 times daily for 3 days.

Refer above to the following remedies. **Camphora, China, Veratrum** and also look at **Arsenicum Album.**

Constipation (Impaction)

This is not very general in pigs and occurs mostly in stall kept animals (too much concentrates) though constipation can be a symptom of another disease or health problem especially liver problems. Insufficient green feed in the ration is usually the cause and you could add bran mashes to the diet to increase the fiber. Make sure the animal has access to lots of water.

Symptoms - Straining and passage of small hard dry lumps of dung which may be covered with slimy mucous, the breath may be foul and the eyes inflamed.

Herbal Treatment

Look to the diet so as to try and find and correct the cause as constipation is more common in stall kept animals. Give a very green and laxative diet and use the following reliable purge for several days. Mix 2 tablespoons of powdered licorice with 1 dessertspoonful of powdered Ginger and add to this 2 ounces of Castor Oil. Mix all together and make paste into round balls. Pulped carrots and parsnips and berry fruits can be added to the diet to help matters. Herbal actions to consider are the Chologogues for bile is the body's natural laxative and the other is Laxative, try to find a herb that covers most of the symptoms. The Bitters are another action to consider as they stimulate peristalsis of the intestines and are good to give to old animals after the initial treatment. Never use liquid paraffin as it demineralizes the body and this could be dangerous for piglets.

Homoeopathic Treatment

Nux Vom 6C - Uncomplicated cases, when there is ingestion of indigestible food. Dose every 2 hours for 3 doses in mild cases. In animals subject to a more chronic condition give a 1M dose night and morning for 2 days.

Sulphur 6C - Abdomen sensitive to pressure and colicky symptoms after drinking. This remedy can most usefully be employed in conjunction with Nux Vom giving the remedies in alternation.

Hydrastis 30C - General catarrhal states, signs of stiffness over lumber region, liver dysfunction and jaundice may be present. Dose 3 times daily for 3 days.

Mag Mur 6C - Liver dysfunction, yellow tongue and other signs of jaundice may appear, stools small and crumbly, Dose 3 times daily for 3 days.

Bryonia 6C - Stools large hard and may contain blood especially in young animals. Dose 3 times daily for 3 days.

Liver Problems

Jaundice

This can occur as a symptom of inflammation of the liver or sluggish function without inflammation maybe from a congested liver. Obstruction of the bile ducts is another obvious cause. The main cause may be a unsuitable diet especially over prolonged use of concentrated unnatural cakes and meals which may of overloaded and congested the liver. Also vermifuges (wormers) may over time damage the liver and produce jaundice. Poisons and poisoning also damages the liver so make sure the animal hasn't been eating anything it shouldn't.

Symptoms - The mucous membranes of the eyes, mouth and nose become tinged with yellow and the skin also shows this discoloration. Urine becomes dark green because of the presence of bile, constipation may be present, faeces is light in color (nearly white if the bile duct is blocked) and in some cases there may be edema of the limbs. Pressure along the margin of the short ribs produces pain, the appetite is poor and the animal shows hardly any inclination to drink (can be the opposite to), the animal lays down much and moves with reluctance , has a tottering gait. Sometimes the animal has a dry painful cough and presents a dull stupefied appearance and there may be foul smelling breath.

Herbal Treatment

It is the derangement of the bile flow which is the basic cause for this complaint and until it is normalized the yellow pigment will continue to be noticeable especially in the eyes. Give a short fast with a non-oily purge (Senna pods, Epsom's Salts). It is very important to make sure the purge is non-oily as oil and fats stimulate the secretion of bile. All fatty foods should be avoided in the diet (no linseed, sunflower etc) also avoid giving pulse foods. Give a abundance of Dandelion in the diet the roots can be grated and included as well. Also recommended are Cleavers and Centaury. The main herbal action to look at here is that of the Chologogues and Hepatics and choose from these herbs that seem to cover most of the symptoms. For Hepatitis it is best to use Milk Thistle just on its own for at least a month for this herb is the main regenerative herb for the liver. Some other herbs to look at are Blue Flag and Speedwell.

Speedwell - Used for jaundice, impure blood, dysentery, gastric insufficiency, cough, asthma etc.

Homoeopathic Treatment

Aconite 30C - Give at the onset of the problem especially if it arises from cold or there is fever.

Berberis Vulgaris 30C - Sluggish liver conditions with tenderness over lumber region. Skin yellowish, urinary symptoms present. Dose 3 times daily for 3 days.

Chelidonium 6C - Pain and tenderness over right shoulder area. Strong yellow discolouration of visible mucous membranes. Obstruction of bile ducts. Dose 3 times daily for 3 days.

China 30C - Weakness and debility, abdominal pain, stools yellow and fluid, increasing weakness. Dose every 3 hours for 4 doses.

Lycopodium 200C - Flatulent state, indifferent appetite, abdominal tympany after eating, mucous membranes greyish yellow and urine loaded with red sediment. Dose night and morning for 5 days.

Mag Mur 30C - Enlargement of liver with difficulty in urination, jaundice and abdominal pain pronounced. Dose night and morning for 4 days.

Herbal Overview of The Digestive System

Unfortunately one of the main ways of diagnosing what sort of disease an animal has is to do an autopsy straight after it has died, this has to be done especially in fast acting diseases that kill fast. Always isolate the animal from the others and clean and disinfect where the animal has been so as to minimize the spread of infection. In dealing with problems of the digestive system it's always best to start with a purge so as to clean the system and bowels out. This is very important especially when you do not know what you are dealing with because you are purging out hopefully most of the toxins that are causing the condition. After the purge isolate and fast the animal for 24 hours and see what happens. Always start on the Garlic and Echinacea straight away as the Echinacea is also used to treat septicemia and to attack blood borne toxins and with Garlic being antiviral and antibacterial we have together a good strong initial attack. If you look at the herbal treatment sections above you will see they cover most of the conditions of the digestive system and should give you helpful information.

Below is a list of Herbal Actions that are used for the digestive system read through them and become familiar with them for in Herbal Medicine you always think in actions needed not the Herb needed this way the mind stays on the big picture.

Herbal Actions for The Digestive System

Anti-biotic - Always start with Garlic as this is both anti-bacterial and anti-viral as well as being used for killing parasites and worms, your initial attack begins here.

Herbs - Echinacea, Garlic, Myrrh, Pau D' Arco, Reshi.

Anti-emetic - Can reduce a feeling of nausea and can help to relieve or prevent vomiting.

Herbs - Cayenne, Fennel, Meadowsweet, Peppermint,

Anti-inflammatory - Helps the body to combat inflammations, there will always be pain, heat and maybe fever when these are called for. Herbs mentioned under demulcents will often act in this way especially when they are applied to coat for example a inflamed intestine or any other inflamed organ.(Slippery Elm).

Herbs - Cranesbill, Chamomile, Eyebright, Feverfew, Ginger, Golden Rod, Ladys Mantle, Licorice, Marshmallow, Meadowsweet, Marigold, Pau D' Arco, Witch Hazel, Wormwood.

Anti-microbial - Helps the body destroy or resist pathogenic micro-organisms.

Herbs - Aniseed, Cayenne, Echinacea, Garlic, Gentian, Marigold, Myrrh, Peppermint, Rosemary, Rue, Sage, Thyme, Wormwood.

Antispasmodic - Prevents or eases spasms and cramps especially of the intestines.

Herbs - Aniseed, Angelica, Chamomile, Fennel, Rosemary, Rue, Sage, Skullcap, St John's Wort, Thyme, Valerian, Vervain.

Anti-viral - Astragalus, Cats claw, Echinacea, Garlic, Myrrh?, Shitake, St John's Wort, Pau D'Arco.

Anthelmintic - Destroys or expels worms from the digestive system.

Herbs - Garlic, Tansy, Wormwood, Thyme, Rue.

Aperient - Mild laxative.

Herbs - Burdock, Dandelion.

Astringent - Contracts tissue which in turn reduces discharges, these herbs contain tannins. In the digestive system they can be used to stop diarrhea and in the treatment of ulcers. Most astringents also have a anti-bacterial action.

Herbs - Agrimony, Bear Berry, Cranesbill, Comfrey, Eyebright, Golden Rod, Hops, Ladys Mantle, Marigold, Marshmallow, Meadowsweet, Nettles, Raspberry, Sage, Rosemary, Slippery Elm, Shepherds Purse, St John's Wort, Slippery Elm, Thyme, Witch Hazel, Yarrow.

Bitters - Herbs that taste bitter act as stimulating tonics for the digestive system.

Herbs -Burdock, Feverfew, Gentian, Hops, Horehound, Rue, Tansy, Wormwood.

Carminative - Stimulates peristalsis of the digestive system and relaxes the stomach and helps remove gas and wind from the system.

These herbs are usually rich in volatile oils.

Herbs - Aniseed, Angelica, Cayenne, Chamomile, Fennel, Garlic, Ginger, Golden Rod, Hyssop, Horseradish, Juniper, Parsley, Peppermint, Penny Royal, Sage, Rosemary, Tansy, Thyme, Valerian, Wormwood.

Cholagogue - Stimulates the release of bile from the gallbladder which can relieve gallbladder problems, bile is also the body's natural laxative so cholagogues have a laxative effect as well.

Herbs - Agrimony, Blue Flag, Dandelion, Fumitory, Gentian, Marigold, Milk Thistle, Yellow Dock.

Demulcent - Soothes and protects irritated or inflamed internal tissues.

Herbs - Bear Berry, Corn Silk, Coltsfoot, Comfrey, Fenugreek, Licorice, Marshmallow, Milk Thistle, Mullein, Oats, Plantain, Slippery Elm.

Diaphoretic - Aids the skin in the elimination of toxins and produces sweat thus reducing the temperature of fevers.

Herbs - Angelica, Black Cohosh, Cayenne, Chamomile, Elder, Elecampane, Fennel, Garlic, Ginger, Golden Rod, Guaiacum, Hyssop, Lime Blossom, Peppermint, Sarsaparilla, Thyme, Vervain, Yarrow.

Hepatic - Tones and strengthens the liver, may increase the flow of bile.

Herbs - Agrimony, Blue Flag, Dandelion, Fennel, Fumitory, Gentian, Horseradish, Hyssop, Motherwort, Milk Thistle, Vervain, Wormwood, Yarrow.

Laxative - Promotes the evacuation of the bowels.

Herbs - Burdock, Dandelion., Fumitory, Horseradish, Licorice,

Parasiticide - Kills parasites and insects.

Herbs - Aniseed, Rosemary,

Sialagogue - Stimulates the secretion of saliva.

Herbs - Blue flag, Cayenne, Gentian, Ginger.

The Nervous System

Encephalitis

This term implies inflammation of the brain or any inflammatory lesion occurring to the brain tissue. It leads to loss of nervous function. Most cases are related to bacterial or viral infection though injury can be a cause.

Symptoms - Encephalitis is usually accompanied by fever, toxemia, anorexia, depression and tachycardia. Normal stimuli can produce exaggerated responses, the animal being easily startled. There may be convulsions accompanied by squinting of eyes and clamping of jaws. Excitement may be a early sign, brain involvement is evident by bellowing, head shaking and staring pupils and maybe head pressing.

Herbal Treatment

Herbal treatment could be too slow for a fast acting disease as this but consider Garlic, Echinacea and Myrrh for bacterial and viral infections. Another herb to look at is St John's Wort because it is a Nervine anti-viral. Essential oils can cross the blood brain barrier and could be a fast way of getting into the area so try maybe Garlic oil ,Lavender oil, Myrrh, Thyme or Eucalyptus diluted and rubbed in the head area as these are all anti microbials. I have not heard of essential oils being used for this condition but as a last desperate resort I would try it. Homoeopathy is the better action to take as it is faster acting then herbal medicine and I would also give Vitamin C injections straight away a 50cc intramuscularly with half the dose on each side of the body. Most vets would give you not much hope.

Homoeopathic Treatment

Aconite 200C - If seen early enough give in the febrile stage. Dose hourly for 4 hours.

Arnica 30C - Give this remedy if the cause of the condition was from injury.

Belladonna 1M - This remedy is useful for deranged nerve conditions, there is a accompanying full bounding pulse, fever, dilated pupils and a smooth hot skin, convulsions, excitement and head pressing. Dose hourly for 4 doses.

Stramonium 30C - Indicated when signs of vertigo appear, such as a tendency to stagger and fall sideways, the eyes are usually wide open and staring. Dose 4 times daily for 2 days.

Hyoscyamus 200C - Indications for this remedy include frequent head shaking and a tendency to muscular twitching. There may be signs of abdominal discomfort. Dose 3 times daily for 3 days.

Phosphorus 200C - Useful in less acute cases showing a tendency to reoccur. The animal becomes unsteady after rising. Dose night and morning for one week.

Zincum Met 6C - Indicated where there is a tendency for the head to roll from side to side. Hyperaesthesia and hyperexcitability are present, easily startled, paddling of feet may occur. Dose 3 times daily for 3 days.

Meningitis

Inflammation of the ménages is usually secondary to viral or bacterial infection. Infection may enter through a penetrating wound but more often the infection is spread through the blood. Usually effects pigs 2 to 8 weeks of age and is fairly rare in adults.

Symptoms - This condition is characterized by fever and muscle rigidity. Restlessness and head shaking are common which can go on to pressing the head against any suitable object. Sensitivity of the skin is a common symptom, there is a retraction of the head and stiffness of the neck muscles, paresis of the hindquarters is common. There can be increased nervous activity and so increased response to pain, excitement or depression and a raised body temperature.

Herbal Treatment

This is the same as Encephalitis. Meningitis is a fast acting acute infection and herbal remedies may act to slow to control the condition but would be very helpful in assisting the recovery.

The best action here is to call the vet and hope they have the right antibiotics to target the cause.

Refer to Encephalitis and use the treatment given there.

Homoeopathic Treatment

Aconite 200C - Should be given in the early febrile stage, the animal usually looks anxious and there is a rapid short pulse. Dose hourly for 4 hours.

Apis 6C - The acute form is sometimes associated with edema of the meninges and this remedy will benefit such cases. Dose every half hour for 5 doses.

Belladonna 1M - The indications for this remedy are a accompanying encephalitis with dilated pupils and a throbbing pulse, the skin is smooth and hot, sweating is common. Dose 2 hourly for 3 doses.

Zincum Met 6C - Indicated where there is a tendency for the head to roll from side to side. Hyperaesthesia and hyper excitability are present, easily startled, paddling of feet may occur. Dose 3 times daily for 3 days.

Bryonia 6C - Indicated in cases showing vertigo, the animal resents movement and there is excessive dryness of the mucous membranes eg seen in the mouth where the lips show a parched appearance and there is great thirst. Dose 3 times daily for 3 days.

Veratum 30C - The legs and ears are icy cold, there is convulsive trembling of the whole body or there is a reeling, staggering motion, the animal plunges violently and falls down head first.

Cuprum Met 30C - A useful remedy when convulsions are associated more with meningitis then with encephalitis. The head usually assumes a lowered posture and there may be attempts to press it against any suitable object.

Tetanus (Lock Jaw)

This disease is caused by the bacterium Clostridium tetani gaining entrance to the body through a puncture or other deep wounds that are not exposed to the air.

Symptoms - The animal walks in a unsteady manner, there is muscle stiffness and muscular spasms. Severe cases involve the central nervous system with convulsions and death from respiratory failure.

Herbal Treatment

The main herb to think of here is Hypericum also known as St Johns Wort. This herb is used as a nervine anti-viral and bacterial. Traditionally it has been used to help prevent tetanus especially in horses that have trodden on a nail that has gone through the fetlock.

The treatment for horses was to pour straight tincture into the wound in the hope it would kill the bacteria. Treat all wounds with Hypericum and Calendula tinctures mixed half and half diluted with water. See the Animal First Aid Book.

Homoeopathic Treatment

The following remedies may give some relief and in mild cases and may lead to cure especially if started early.

Acconitum 10M - For the fear and anxiety, always give at the first signs of a problem. Give every hour for 4 doses.

Curare 30C - Helps where muscle stiffness is prominent. Give three times daily for 7days.

Strychninum 200C - The arching of the back together with extension of limbs and head matches the symptoms of this remedy. Give twice daily for 3 days.

Hypericum 1M - This remedy may help in limiting the spread of the toxin. Give three times daily for 7 days.

Ledum 6C - This is the main remedy for puncture wounds especially if they feel cold. Give frequently in the potency.

Tetanus Nosode - Combine the nosode with the selected remedy. Use for 7 days in the 30th potency.

Herbal Overview Of The Nervous System

One of the most important herbs in this system is Hypericum also known as St Johns Wort. This herb is anti-viral, antibacterial, anti-inflammatory, a sedative and one of our main first aid remedies for wounds which helps relieve pain and can kill the tetanus bacteria and this is only mentioning a part of its uses, always consider this when there are problems with this system especially if you don't know what the problem is. Another good herb for rebuilding this system is Oats which is a Nervine tonic also think of Valerian which is our main Tranquilliser but also a good tonic for this system. A lot of the herbs mentioned below are used in a lot of other body systems as well so when you want the action of a Nervine to use in another system try to match the herb to one used in that system as well.

Antispasmodic - Prevents or eases spasms and cramps.

Herbs - Aniseed, Angelica, Black Cohosh, Chamomile, Fennel,

Horehound, Hyssop, Lime Blossom, Mistletoe, Motherwort, Rosemary, Rue, Sage, Skullcap, St johns Wort, Thyme, Valerian, Vervain.

Nervine - Has a beneficial effect on the nervous system, acts like a tonic to this system.

Herbs - Black Cohosh, Chamomile, Hops, Lime Blossoms, Mistletoe, Motherwort, Oats, Peppermint, Rosemary, Skullcap, St Johns Wort, Tansy, Thyme, Valerian, Vervain, Wormwood.

Sedative - Calms the nervous system and reduces stress and nervousness throughout the body.

Herbs - Black Cohosh, Chamomile, Hops, Hyssop, Motherwort, Skullcap, St Johns Wort, Valerian , Vervain.

Notes

The Urinary System

Acute Nephritis   (Inflammation of the Kidney)

This condition is rarely seen by itself there is usually a cause such as Septicemic infections which are brought to the kidney by the blood. The condition may also arise as a sequel to mastitis, metritis or some other septic condition. Chemical poisoning frequently leads to Nephritis. Another pathway to consider is that of a bladder infection that has traveled up the ureters to the kidney.

Symptoms - There is a initial rise in temperature with accelerated pulse followed by anorexia and possibly increased respiration. Tenderness over the kidney area is common, the urine itself may contain blood, pus, mucous and proteins may be present.

The pig may stand with the back arched and the hind legs extended backwards and outwards and there may be frequent urination of small amounts of highly colored urine with maybe occasional difficulty in passing. When made to move the patient does so with hesitation and groaning especially if turned in a narrow circle.

Herbal Treatment

The first thing to do here is to try and establish the cause and remove that. After using Garlic and Echinacea (blood borne toxins) think of the herbs Parsley, Chicory, Golden Rod and Chaparral. Other herbs to consider for kidney problems are Bearberry, Buchu and Corn silk. Remember this is a life threatening problem and a vet should be called because there may have to be some very quick decisions made. Actions to consider here are the Anti-inflammatorys, Alteratives which are the blood cleansers along with the Demulcents which should work with the anti-inflammatorys so as to reduce the pain. Think also of the urinary antiseptics so as to stop the infection from taking up residence down the line.

Homoeopathic Treatment

Apis 6C - Renal edema in the acute form, urine shows albuminous casts. Dose every 2 hours for 4 doses.

Arsenicum 1M - Scanty urine showing albumen content and drops of blood, the animal is restless   and thirsty for small amounts, there is a harsh dry coat, symptoms are worse after midnight. Dose every 3 hours for 4 doses.

Belladonna 1M - Acute cases showing excitement and dilated pupils, full bounding pulse and hot smooth skin, straining to pass urine which is scanty and loaded with phosphates, blood in urine is common. Dose every 2 hours for 4 doses.

Beberis 6C - Tenderness over the kidneys and sacral region accompanies frequent urination, the urine is cloudy and contains a reddish sediment. Dose 3 hourly for 4 doses.

Mercurius Sol 30C - Urine scanty with greenish mucous sediment which may contain pus and blood. Urine is dark colored. Dose 3 times daily for 4 days.

Lycopodium 200C - Urine profuse during the night, tendency to retention with thick reddish sediment. Dose night and morning for 5 days.

Phosphorus 200C - Acute cases showing blood in urine, blood is diffused throughout the urine giving a brownish appearance. Dose night and morning for 3 days.

Nat Mur 200C - Chronic cases showing a pale urine of low specific gravity, there is usually salt retention leading to thirst and anemia. Dose night and morning for one week.

Urolithiasis - (Stones and Gravel)

This condition may arise from too heavily mineralized bore water and stasis of the urine. Various factors contribute including dry feeding and lack of water. A study of the makeup of a passed stone may give you a clue as to the cause of the problem.

Symptoms - Obvious difficulty in passing urine which is scanty and blood stained. Signs of pain include kicking at belly and looking around at flanks. Severe attacks are called renal colic and this may be shown by frequent uneasy shifting of the hind limbs, shaking or twisting of the tail, looking around at the flanks and lying down and rising again at short intervals without apparent cause. In bad cases inflammation of the kidneys may set in. There can be lots of complications with stones with some of the worst being blocked ureters which are between the kidney and bladder and then there may be a blockage after the bladder as is common in males.

Herbal Treatment

The same treatment as for kidney disorders should be followed but first try and establish the cause. Couch grass should always be added to the Parsley or any of the other herbs given for the cure of Nephritis. Warm milk and molasses is highly beneficial for this complaint fortified with Slippery Elm Bark (one heaped tablespoon full to the quart). Also look at the herbs Cleavers, Bearberry, Gravel Root and Chaparral which all have the action of antilithics. Horsetail is another good herb for stones as it is high in silica and this may help to break up the stone. It is also wise to add some demulcents to sooth the pain caused by gravel scraping its way down, some good ones for this system are Corn silk and Marshmallow. Pat Coleby says if the problem is from highly mineralized water add a little apple cider vinegar in the food and stones do not occur. The amount needed is surprisingly small, just a desert spoon every few days would be enough. Two teaspoons full can also be given daily for two or three days as it may help dissolve the stones and flush the bits out. Prevention is better than cure.

Homoeopathic Treatment - See also cystitis

Lycopodium 200C - Hepatic symptoms with blood stained urine containing red sediment, the early stages of stone formation. Dose night and morning for 7 days.

Sarsaparilla 6C - Pain at the beginning and end of urination especially at the end, Urine contains gravely deposits and is slimy. Dose 3 times daily for 3 days.

Urtica Urens 6X - Thickens the urine and removes the tendency to gravel formation by removing the basic salts that help form it, it will also increase the quantity of urine passed, there may be a skin rash, give one dose 3 times daily for 10 days.

Calc Phos 30C - A good constitutional remedy which will help regulate the calcium and phosphate metabolism and so prevent the formation of phosphates, it should be given as a routine remedy in young animals up till the age of one. One dose weekly for 8 weeks.

Mag Mur 6C - May help in preventing some forms of stones and may be given as a routine remedy if the urine shows suspicious deposits and there are other signs of stone formation.

Cystitis

Inflammation of the bladder can arise from a infection in some other part of the urinary system and a infection here can also travel up the ureters and infect the kidneys if not looked after. Cystitis can also arise as a result of stones and gravel damaging the delicate tissue and leaving it open for infection. This condition can be acute or chronic with the acute condition usually caused by bacteria and the chronic caused by gravel and stones. This condition is seldom seen in young pigs. Another common cause is difficult birthing leading to a infection especially from poor hygiene.

Symptoms - Frequent urination is the commonest sign with the urine often containing blood. There may be considerable difficulty in passing urine. Arching of the back and signs of pain are evident such as kicking at the abdomen and urinating while lying down. There may be constant tail wagging as if on heat and there could be swelling of the vulva.

Herbal Treatment

The main herbs we use in cystitis are the urinary antiseptics with the best ones being Bearberry and Buchu. Cranberry juice is a good urinary antiseptic as it lines the pipes and prevents bacteria from adhering to them. To the antiseptics we add demulcents which sooth the irritated tissues with the best one for this condition being Corn Silk. You could add to the formula Gravel Root and Chaparral if you think the cause of the condition could be from urinary stones or gravel which tend to scratch and inflame the pipelines leaving them open to infection. Other herbs to consider are Angelica, Yarrow, Agrimony, Cleavers, Damiana, Golden Rod, Juniper, Plantain and Shepherds Purse. These herbs can be mixed as tinctures and then have water added to bring them up to a cup size drench or could be mixed together in dry form and then made into a tea.

Homoeopathic Treatment.

Aconite 30C - In the early febrile involvement when pulse and respiration are increased, frequent ineffectual and painful attempts to urinate, pain on pressure of bladder. Dose every hour for 4 doses.

Cantharis 30C - Much straining and scanty amounts of bloody urine, there is hyperexcitability and signs of sexual irritability, signs of abdominal pain prominent. Dose night and morning in chronic cases for one week, in acute cases give one dose every hour for 4 doses.

Colocynthis 1M - Arching of the back and kicking at the abdomen suggest this remedy. Signs of severe pain are present. Dose every hour for 4 doses.

Nux Vom 30C - When ineffectual urging is associated with digestive upsets. Good to use if Cantharis does not work. Dose 3 times daily for 2 days.

Dulcamara 30C - Catarrhal cystitis resulting from exposure to cold or damp, urine contains a thick mucus or purulent sediment. Dose 3 times daily for 3 days.

Causticum 30C - A useful remedy in the recurrent or chronic form and is especially adapted to the older animal. Follows well after Cantharis which may be needed if acute symptoms flare up in the chronic form.

Uva Ursi 3X - Useful in chronic cystitis, urine is slimy, pain and straining are common. Dose 3 times daily for 7 days.

Herbal Overview of The Urinary System

Most infections get to the kidneys via the blood for the kidneys are the main filter of the blood removing wastes and water. Other infections can start off as cystitis and travel up the ureter and infect the kidney that way so you must always consider both ways. Always ask yourself is the infection traveling from the kidney down or the bladder up? If you think it is the kidney put a leash on the animal and walk them in tight circles one way and then the other. If the animal complains it is probably the kidney. Urinary antiseptics are good for this system whether for treating infection or preventing it as in cases of stones scraping the sides as they go down leaving a wound ripe for infection. Also think of Cranberry for this system as it coats the pipes and stops bacteria getting a foot hold literally.

Herbal Actions For The Urinary System

Anti-biotic - Chaparral, Echinacea, Garlic, Myrrh, Pau D' Arco.

Anti-inflammatory - Helps the body to combat inflammations.

Herbs - Cats Claw, Chaparral, Cleavers, Cranesbill, Eyebright, Ginger, Golden Rod, Guaiacum, Licorice, Marshmallow, Pau D' Arco.

Anti-lithic - Prevent the formation of stones or gravel in the urinary system and helps the body to remove them.

Herbs - Bearberry, Corn Silk, Chaparral, Gravel Root, Horsetail.

Anti-microbial - Helps the body destroy or resist pathogenic micro-organisms.

Herbs - Echinacea, Garlic, Juniper, Myrrh,

Astringent - Contracts tissue which in turn reduces discharges, these herbs contain tannins.

Herbs - Agrimony, Cranesbill, Chaparral, Golden Rod, Horsetail, Shepherds Purse.

Cystitis - Agrimony, Bearberry, Buchu, Celery Seed, Corn Silk, Gravel Root, Golden Rod, Horsetail, Plantain,

Demulcent - Soothes and protects irritated or inflamed internal tissues.

Herbs - Bearberry, Corn Silk, Licorice, Marshmallow, Plantain, Slippery Elm.

Diuretic - Increases the secretion and elimination of urine.

Herbs - Agrimony Angelica, Bear Berry, Blue Flag, Burdock, Buchu, Broom, Coltsfoot, Chaparral, Corn Silk, Dandelion Leaves, Elder, Fumitory, Golden Rod, Guaiacum, Gravel Root, Hawthorn, Horseradish, Horsetail, Juniper, Lime Blossom, Nettles, Pau D' Arco, Penny Royal, Plantain, Parsley, Shepherds Purse, Sarsaparilla, Yarrow.

Urinary Antiseptics - These herbs have a antiseptic action as they pass through the system.

Herbs - Angelica, Bearberry, Buchu, Corn Silk, Golden Rod, Shepherds Purse, Yarrow.

The Muscular Skeletal System

Myositis

Inflammation of the muscle tissue may have its origin in a open wound or infection, or it may be the result of severe straining.

Symptoms - Local heat in the muscle is a early sign, followed by stiffness or lameness if leg muscles are involved. Febrile signs will accompany infectious conditions.

Herbal Treatment

If the cause is from bacterial infection then we would use our immune boosting herbs so as to start fighting the infection, these are Echinacea, Myrrh and Garlic. If inflammation is present treat with anti-inflammatories especially the ones that are pain killers - Willow bark and Devils Claw. If the inflammation was caused by injury try some of the First Aid remedies such as a compress of Arnica Lotion or if the wound is open use Calendula with Hypericum diluted with water as a lotion.

Don't forget to look at the Homoeopathic First Aid remedies.

Homoeopathic Treatment.

Arnica 30C - Should always be given in the early inflammatory stage. Dose again after 2 hours.

Apis 6C - Give if oedema accompanies inflammation. Dose every 3 hours for 4 doses.

Rhus Tox 6C - When the animal gains relief from movement even though the initial movement is painful, symptoms may be more on the left side of the body then the right, indicated when severe wetting or prolong dampness is associated with the onset of the symptoms.

Bryonia 30C - Movement is resented when Bryonia is indicated. The animal will seek to lie on the affected muscles because pressure on them gives ease, warmth is usually useful also.

Hepar Sulph 30C - Infection from a open scratch or wound. Dose 3 times daily for 3 days.

Osteoarthritis

This is a degenerative joint disease of a non-inflammatory origin where the articular cartilages become eroded and bony exostoses that occur at the margin of the joints. All though age plays a part there can be other causes such as systemic or metabolic disturbances. Progressive mild inflammation in the joint over a period of time is more likely to produce osteoarthritis than any other predisposing factor. Osteoarthritis particularly affects the load bearing bones of the body. Being overweight adds to the wear and tear of the joints. Once the cartilage degenerates the cushioning effect is lost within the joint and the joint capsule now becomes involved and the situation becomes worse.

Symptoms - Lameness is the main sign and it could involve several joints. Constant running on concrete and inattention to hooves which can become overgrown can cause arthritis. In older animals with arthritis the joints may join together, especially the neck and elbow joints and the animal may walk with a stilted action and the neck may be extended as that of a tortoise.

Herbal Treatment

Nutrition wise for the early stages you can give calcium, Vitamin D, magnesium and manganese so as to try to stop the condition from getting worse this is of course after you have checked to see if the diet and too much calcium was the cause. Glucosamine and Chondroitin Sulphate can help stimulate the rebuilding of cartilage and help in the early stages of arthritis.

Arthritis with lots of pain and inflammation needs the use of the anti-inflammatory herbs; good ones to use for this condition are Meadowsweet, Devils Claw and Willow Bark as these act as good pain killers as well. Other herbs to use are the alteratives which clean out the area and the system some good ones are Burdock, Garlic, Sarsaparilla and Chaparral which has a antioxidant action as well. Diuretic herbs are also used for this condition as they help to remove the metabolic waste and toxins which usually result from the constant inflammation and help the kidneys flush this waste out, some good ones are Celery seed, Juniper (these two are best used together) and Dandelion leaf. Celery Seed is a good acid remover so this action alone could help a lot. Other herbs to look at for arthritis are Black Cohosh, Cats Claw, Guaiacum, Nettles, Wild Yam and Yellow dock. Add Licorice to the formula at about 10% as this will help in the assimilation of the formula into the body.

Homoeopathic Treatment

Not an easy condition to treat. Start treatment as early as possible so as to slow down deterioration. Useful remedies for the early inflammatory stages are.

Rhus Tox 6C - This remedy is indicated when the animal's symptoms are eased after a short period of movement there may be initial stiffness on first moving.

Bryonia 6C - The indications for this remedy are the opposite of the above, the animal prefers to remain still and any movement causes distress and sometimes acute pain evidenced by the animal crying out.

Calc Flour 30C - May be needed in the latter stages once the exostoses and joint swellings develop. The carpus is the main joint affected when this remedy is indicated. There may be accompanying cystic tumours around the joint.

Rhus Tox 1M - This can be given in the latter stages to help with the symptoms of pain when the animal moves.

Arthritis Due To Infection

There are 3 main diseases that can lead to arthritis in pigs they are Mycoplasma hyorinis, Haemophilus parasuis and Erysipelothrix rhusiopathiae. This condition can also be caused by pyogenic bacteria getting in the joint mainly from injury the main organisms are Streptococci and Staphylococci.

Symptoms - There may be a initial temperature rise and febrile signs may develop. The affected joint becomes swollen, stiff, tense and hot due to inflammation. Pain is obvious by the onset of severe lameness. Examination may reveal the presence of punctures on the skin and the appearance of a purulent exudate.

Herbal Treatment

For this condition think of our infection fighting herbs such as Echinacea, Garlic and Myrrh. If the skin is broken and you think the infection got in this way apply a lotion or cream of Calendula and Hypericum to the area. To our infection fighting herbs you can add some of the anti-inflammatories, alteratives and diuretics that are mentioned in Osteo-Arthritis. Add Licorice to the formula at about 10% as this will help in the assimilation of the formula into the body.

Homoeopathic Treatment

Aconitum 30C - This should be given as soon as possible in the early febrile stage.

Ferrum Phos 6C - This also is a good remedy for the initial feverish stage more often indicated when throat symptoms accompany the invasive process.

Belladonna 30C - Indicated when the patient presents a excitable picture with dilated pupils, throbbing arteries and a hot skin.

Bryonia 6C - Symptoms worse for movement, relief from pain on pressure over the joint and a possible involvement with the respiratory tract. The joint is usually extremely hard and tense.

Apis Mel 6C - If the synovial sheaf of the joint becomes edematous indicated by swelling this remedy may help. The patient is made worse by heat in any form and does not drink much.

Ledum 6C - The remedy of choice if the arthritis has been caused by the penetration of a sharp object giving rise to a puncture wound.

Iodum 6C - This is a remedy which sometimes gives good results in the less acute case especially when the joint pains are worse at night. The patient is often thin with a voracious appetite and the skin is dry and withered looking.

Rhus Tox 6C - The indications for this remedy is relief from movement although there may be initial stiffness on rising. Maybe accompanying skin symptoms of a vesicular itchy nature.

Silica 30C - This remedy is indicated in the more chronic case. There may be involvement of neighboring lymphatic glands showing cold abscesses.

Degenrative Jiont Disease (Osteochondrosis)

This is a common disease that affects young growing pigs causing lameness and joint deformities. The cause is more from breeding with the end result being a heavy long pig with short legs. These short legs now have to support a large body so they are prone to damage and wear and tear.

Symptoms - The largest pigs in the litter are the main candidates for this condition. Look for lameness and favoring of a limb. Limb deformities begin in young pigs but the clinical problems are not noticed till about 4 to 8 months of age. Clinical signs vary with the site and the extent of the damage but can range from stiffness and a shortened stride to a angular deformity of a leg.

Herbal Treatment - Sometimes deficiencies of zinc and manganese have been indicated in this condition and also treatment for metabolic acidosis has had some success to. Have a good look at what is mentioned in Osteoarthritis. For treating acidosis cut down the protein intake as this breaks down to uric acid. Consider the Herbs Celery Seed (the acid remover) and Meadowsweet (the acid balancer). I would consider giving a good human calcium bio supplement with calc, mag, D, Horsetail (silica) and boron for strengthening the surface of the bones. Consider also diet, what if you kept them fairly lean and light while young and fatten the up after maturity when the bones have finished growing.

Homoeopathic Treatment

Calc Phos 30C - This is our main remedy especially in the young. Helps to stabilize the mineral balance and produce strong bones and muscles. Dose 3 times per week for 4 weeks.

Helca Lave 200C - May help in hardening the bones and may help in preventing the condition from getting worse. Dose 3 times per week for 4 weeks.

Silica 200C - May also help in the hardening of the bones and works well with Calc Phos. Dose 3 times per week for 6 weeks.

Broken Leg

With pigs having such short legs its fairly hard to break them and if this does happen take into consideration the diet especially the Calc, Mag and Boron mineral intake also consider how much weight there is on the body. Make some wooden splints and bandage them firmly (not tightly allow for expansion from swelling) to the leg once you have set the leg. Another good alternative is to use a plastic pipe cut in half down the center then cut the top and bottom to size. Line with cotton wool or foam and use as a splint. Use an elastic type of bandage and observe because with fractures the leg can swell and if the bandages are tight circulation will be cut off. If there are lacerations with the fracture you could make a lotion from Comfrey and Calendula together and soak the cotton wool with this. Be careful if you use wood that it doesn't swell and tighten the bandage. Fast the animal and observe for one or 2 days giving a Comfrey Brew night and morning. Give the appropriate Homoeopathics below pays special attention to Arnica and Ledum so as to reduce the swelling and internal bleeding fast.

Homoeopathic Treatment

Arnica 6C- For the shock and bruised sore pains. Arnica cream can also be applied as long as the skin is not broken.

Calc Phos 6X - Helps in nutrition especially of the bones and promotes the knitting together of the bones. Helps fractures heal much faster. Can be used in alternation with Symphytum.

Ledum 6C- Take after arnica 4 hourly or 3 times a day to assist in the absorption of the extravasation of blood after a fracture so as to reduce the swelling which may take up to 3 to 4 days. Helps to absorb the internal bleeding after a fracture.

Symphytum 6C - More commonly known as comfrey or knitbone or bone set. The names says it all. Promotes fast healing of bones, use with Calc Phos 6X. Take both 3 times daily till better.

Herbal Overview - The Muscular Skeletal System

For bruising think about Arnica in a lotion and use the Homoeopathic dose internally, for broken bones think about Comfrey as its old name is knit bone. For arthritis and rheumatism use your Anti Rheumatics, Anti-Inflammatorys, Analgesics but also think of Celery Seed as this is called the acid remover and another herb to think of is Meadowsweet as this herb is called the acid balancer. It is usually the high acid in the system that irritates the joints and starts the inflammation so these 2 herbs could remove the cause for the condition; also consider diet as a diet high in protein will create a lot of acid waste. For blood borne bacterial infections think of the Alteratives (blood cleansers) and Anti Bacterials especially our main ones Garlic and Echinacea. If there is damage to the joints use a nutritional supplement with these 3 together - Glucosamine Sulphate,

Chondroitin and MSM as these together will help rebuild the joints.

Herbal Actions for The Muscular Skeletal System

Alterative - Herbs that gradually restore proper function to the body, they increase health and vitality. They were once known as the blood cleansers.

Herbs - Black Cohosh, Blue Flag, Burdock, Chaparral, Echinacea, Garlic, Nettles, Pau D'Arco ,Sarsaparilla, Yellow Dock.

Analgesic - Herbs that reduce pain.

Herbs - Black Cohosh, Chamomile, Hops, Meadowsweet, Pau D'Arco, Peppermint, Skullcap, St John's Wort, Valerian.

Anti-biotic - Chaparral, Echinacea, Garlic, Myrrh, Pau D' Arco.

Antispasmodic - Prevents or eases spasms and cramps.

Herbs - Angelica, Black Cohosh, Chamomile, Skullcap, St John's Wort, Valerian.

Anti-inflammatory - Helps the body to combat inflammations.

Herbs - Cats Claw, Devils Claw, Chaparral , Feverfew, Ginger, Guaiacum, Licorice, Meadowsweet, Pau D' Arco, Sarsaparilla, St John's Wort, Willow Bark.

Anti-viral - Astragalus, Cats claw, Echinacea, Garlic, Myrrh?, St John's Wort, Pau D'Arco.

Anti-Rheumatic - Angelica, Burdock, Black Cohosh, Chaparral, Cats Claw, Celery Seed, Dandelion, Garlic, Guaiacum, Nettles, Willow Bark, Yellow Dock.

Rubefacient - Causes a gentle local irritation to the skin which stimulates the capillaries to open increasing the blood flow.

Herbs - Cayenne, Garlic, Ginger, Horseradish, Nettles, Peppermint Oil, Rosemary Oil, Rue.

Notes

The Skin

Foot Rot

Foot Rot is a bacterial infection and in pigs it is often found to be the Fusiformis necrophorus strain which is the same one that causes the condition in sheep. This condition can develop at any age but concrete floors may increase the incidence in the young. There can be a lot of problems with secondary infections and neglected cases can lead to septicemia. In some places notification of this disease in compulsory.

Symptoms - Slight lameness is the early sign often in just a single limb with extreme lameness showing a severe condition. Cracks develop on the wall of the hoof and the condition develops gradually with the foot becoming swollen. Lesions vary in severity and can include heel erosions, separation along the white line, toe erosions, sole erosions, deep necrotic ulcers and sinuses at the coronary band. Secondary infections can lead to ulceration of certain areas which can become deep and may damage bones and tendons.

Prevention - Disinfect flooring. Foot baths with copper sulphate and formalin. Also never put a new animal straight into the herd always quarantine for a while. If animals have to be kept in damp areas inspect feet regularly.

Herbal Treatment - The presence of foot rot indicates that the land is not well. Diet wise Juliette de Bairacli Levy recommends a purge and then build up the animals on with good natural foods. Dose animals with Garlic and Echinacea. For area treatment wash in a bath of mild detergent with disinfectant and lots of salt added. After area is clean inspect and trim hooves carefully. Bathe with a lotion of calendula and Hypericum. Hypericum (St John's Wort) in this case should help pain. Apply a cream to the area made up of Calendula and Hypericum. Do this twice each day and give the Homoeopathic remedies indicated. Keep animals in a dry clean sick bay for a few days so you can monitor progress. I would be inclined to keep the lotion in a spray bottle and spray the feet every time I walked past.

Homoeopathic Treatment

Kreosotum 200C- This is one of the main remedies as it has a profound action on diseased horn and surrounding tissues. Give twice weekly for 4 to 6 weeks.

Hepar Sulph 1M - The pain associated with the condition should be relieved by this remedy. Give daily for seven days.

Silicea 200C - Once the acute state has been relieved follow on with this remedy as it will quickly build up hard healthy horn which will more easily resist subsequent reinfection. Give twice weekly for 6 weeks.

Pyrogen 1M - If septicemia develops this is the remedy to use. Dose 3 times daily for 3 days.

Foot Rot Nosode - A 30C potency of the nosode should be given at the beginning of autumn and then again in spring twice weekly for 6 weeks. This should hopefully act as a preventative. In acute conditions give daily with the selected remedy for 7 days.

Ringworm

Ringworm lesions in pigs are caused by the fungal agents Microsporum and Trichophyton. This condition is a fungal infection that is highly contagious between animals and can be passed on to humans. Diseases which can be mistaken for ringworm are greasy pig, pityriasis rosea and sarcoptic mange.

Symptom - Reddish circular lesions appear on the skin especially in the abdominal area and latter progress to a dry scabby lesion. Other common areas are behind the ears and the back of the neck. They first appear as brownish nodules that enlarge and join together to form a large roughened area with dry crusts around the edges. Unusually in pigs there is no itching or hair loss.

Herbal Treatment

Ringworm is a fungal infection which usually attacks when the immune system is weakened by stress or exhaustion. Fungi thrive in damp, dark and confined places. If you think the immune system is run down you can give Echinacea, zinc, and vitamin C and you might as well give garlic as this has an anti-fungal action. Externally treatment can be a lotion of calendula 1 to 5 in strength for cleaning the area and around it. Stronger anti-fungals may be necessary as this can sometimes be a very stubborn condition to get rid of. Garlic is a stronger anti-fungal and you can use this externally and internally at the same time. Another strong anti-fungal we have is Tea Tree oil which can be put on neat to the infected area. Other herbs that have been traditionally used for this condition are Herb Robert, Lemon juice, Rue and Walnut.

Treatment

Raise immunity.

Calendula lotion 1 to 5 strength on and around the affected area. (can mix with garlic)

Tea tree oil - strong anti-fungal dab on to the affected area neat.

Garlic externally on effected area and latter if problem is not resolving take internally.

Raw lemon juice applied twice daily.

Other herbs to look at are Burdock, Elder, Sarsaparilla, Myrrh and Rue.

Homoeopathic Treatment

Bacillinum 200C - This nosode has a proven record in the treatment of ringworm. 2 doses at two week intervals with sepia 6C.

Sepia 200C - Use with the above remedy in bad out breaks and by itself in mild outbreaks. Dose once per week for 4 weeks.

Tellurium 30C - Twice a day for one week especially when lesions tend to be equally distributed on either side of the body.

Chrysarobinum 6C - 3 times a day for 5 days, when the disease has progressed to the crusty stage.

Note - Animals that are susceptible to ringworms are usually deficient in copper. Give a Kelp Supplement.

Pityriasis Rosea

Also known as Porcine Juvenile Pustular Psoriaform Dermatitis. The cause of this disease is unknown and it can affect young pigs from 2 weeks to 10 months of age. The disease is mild and recovery can be expected in 6 to 8 weeks. Usually only odd pigs develop the condition but it is possible for entire litters to get it. The disease is considered to be partly heredity as the Landrace breed of pigs is the most effected.

Symptoms - The skin lesions are reddish papules which are hot to the touch, the lesions enlarge at their periphery and lesions close by may join together. The center of the lesion is flat and covered with a bran like scale overlaying the normal skin. The lesions are mainly on the abdomen but are occasionally seen on the back, neck and legs. As in ringworm there is again no itching.

Herbal Treatment - Treat the same as Ringworm. Hypericum has a antiviral action so with Calendulas antibacterial and anti-fungal action we are covering most of the bases. Use Tea Tree oil in a test area and see what happens.

Homoeopathic Treatment

Sulphur 30C - Lesions are red and look wet, worse for warmth. Dose night and morning for 5 days.

Petroleum 200C - Blistery eruptions with tendency to suppuration of cracked skin which bleeds easily, skin usually dry. Dose night and morning for 1 week.

Mezereum 200C - Has given good results in similar cases especially when back lesions are dominate. Dose daily for 7 days.

Greasy Pig

This disease is also known as Exudative Epidermitis. The cause of the condition is the bacteria Staph. hyicus which seems unable to penetrate unbroken skin but gets into the system through cuts and wounds. Older pigs develop a resistance to this disease. 5 to 60 day old pigs are the main target of the infection which can lead to dehydration and death. There can be a high death rate in this disease. High Humidity is associated with severe outbreaks.

Symptoms - This disease has a sudden onset. The first signs are listlessness and the development of a reddish or coppery colored skin and the skin becomes covered in reddish brown spots which gradually increase in number and size and take on a damp oily appearance due to the leakage of serum. The skin may thicken and brown scales appear on the groin and axillae which are greasy in texture. The body is rapidly covered with a greasy exudate of sebum and serum that becomes crusty. Sometimes the accumulation of dirt gives the affected area a black color. Affected pigs become depressed and refuse to eat though they may be very thirsty. The temperature may be increased in the early stage of the disease but is near normal in the latter stages. The skin is hot and the coat becomes matted. The eyes may form exudates and discharges. Ulcers appear in the mouth. The hooves may separate from the horn of the heels. Lack of appetite and dehydration may accompany these signs. Yellowish skin is a common feature in milder cases. Recovery can be slow and growth is retarded. In acute cases death can occur in 3 to 5 days. In adult pigs the disease is milder and shows lesions on the back and flanks.

Herbal Treatment - Separate and fast the animal giving Garlic and Echinacea immediately. Echinacea is important here because of it action of attacking strep and staph infections traveling through the blood as well as its action in boosting the immunes system. Pau D arco is another herb to consider.

As this disease can be a killer I would also consider large doses of Vitamin C and maybe even Troys injectable vitamin C. As the pigs become dirty and greasy consider bathing them. Medicate the bath water with Eucalyptus oil and or Tea Tree oil and use soap to wash them. After a wash you can use a lotion of Calendula on the worst areas mixed with Hypericum if you think there is pain. If ulcers appear on the mouth use the Calendula lotion there as well and also consider giving externally.

Homoeopathic Treatment

Morgan Bach 30C - This nosode is well proven in the treatment of skin diseases. Dose daily for 7 days.

Sulphur 200C - A good all round remedy in skin conditions. Dose every week for 3 weeks.

Graphites 30C - If the lesions are more commonly in the groin and axilla areas especially if they have a sticky discharge. Dose 3 time a day for 5 days.

Pulsatilla 30C - Indicated in those conditions that effect the eyes. Dose 3 times daily for 5 days.

Borax 6C - Indicated for the conditions with mouth ulcers. Dose 3 times daily for 7 days.

Silica 200C - Indicated in the conditions where the feet are involved especially the horn. Give 1 dose 3 times per week for 4 weeks.

Cheildonium 30C - Indicated in the conditions where the pigs get a yellow skin. Dose 3 times daily for 7 days.

Swine Pox

This is a viral disease specific to pigs and is different though similar to the other pox diseases. The course of the disease runs from 3 to 4 weeks with a week's incubation period and is a acute often mild infectious disease. This is a vesicular and pustular disease characterized by eruptions of the skin. The disease is frequently seen in young pigs 3 to 6 weeks old but all ages may be affected. Swine Pox is easily transmitted from animal to animal with lice and mites being a fast spreader. Recovered pigs are immune.

Symptoms - The main symptoms are small red areas seen most frequently on the face, ears, abdomen and inside of the legs that develop into papule spots that turn into watery blisters, then to sticky and encrusted scabs (like Chicken Pox) latter dark scabs form which eventually drop or are rubbed off and do not leave a scar. The early stage of the disease may be accompanied by a mild fever. Young piglets are more severely affected then mature pigs and may have lesions all over the body. Older pigs show lesions mainly on the hairless parts of the body and sows may get lesions on the udder and vulva. There may be swelling of the lymph glands in some cases.

Herbal Treatment

Give a short fast. Internal dosing with Garlic and Echinacea. Think of using Astragalus here for its antiviral action. Externally wash the area with a lotion of Calendula and Hypericum or Elder flowers and leaves brewed with garlic.

Pat Coleby says this condition strikes only when the Goat (worth trying for pigs) is deficient in copper. An exterior treatment is a copper and cider vinegar wash which helps the scabs dry up and drop off. Give a copper supplement internally. To make the wash mix a tablespoon of Copper Sulphate with the same amount of Vinegar and mix with 500mls of water this can then be administered with a garden spray bottle and the scabs should start to dry up and drop off.

Homoeopathic Treatment

The following remedies may cut short the infective process and prevent secondary infections.

Antimonium Crud 6C - This remedy is associated with typical papular and pustular skin lesions especially with a generally dry skin. Signs of indigestion may be present. Dose 3 times daily for 3 days.

Cuprum Aceticum 6C - A leading remedy for pox like eruptions frequently accompanied by cramps and spasms of groups of muscles. Diarrhea may also be present. Dose 3 times daily for 3 days.

Kali Bich 30C - The pustules assume a crater like form with yellowish discharge. Dose 2 times daily for 5 days.

Ranunculus Bulbosus 6C - Another useful remedy for the vesicular stage especially if more prominent on the udder. Dose 3 times daily for 5 days.

Calc Flour 30C - This may benefit pigs showing swelling of the lymph glands. Dose daily for 10 days.

Variolinum 30C - This nosode will be found of value either by its self or used in conjunction with the mentioned remedies. Dose daily for 3 days.

Prevention - Give the above nosode on a herd basis. You could make the nosode yourself from the fluid from the weeping pox.

Mange

Caused by the mite Sarcoptes scabiee suis, sarcoptic mange is the only form of any importance in pigs. The mite burrows into the skin to lay eggs. Mites are usually introduced into the herd by a new comer and spread after contact is usually rapid. If commercial applications are used a colony of mites usually survives in the pigs ear hidden away from the sun and chemicals, and it is usually a sow and reinfection starts again through her piglets. Survival of the mite egg away from the host is limited.

Symptoms - Lesions usually start on the head especially the ears and then spread over the body, tail and legs. Itching is usually intense and associated with a hypersensitivity to the mites. As the hypersensitivity subsides the skin is covered with grayish crusts. Itching is the main symptom.

Herbal Treatment

This is a very hard and stubborn condition to treat. A pig with mange requires a preliminary all over washing with lots of soap and warm water to which a little soda, Tea Tree Oil and Eucalyptus Oil has been added (don't forget inside the ears) followed by a thorough cleansing with a hose before any curative treatment can be applied. Herbs used externally for this condition are Garlic, Rue, Wormwood, and Neem. A small portion of ammonia can be added to the external preparations or you could add 50% vinegar. Lemon juice has also traditionally been used for mange. Dose the animal internally with garlic and Wormwood.

Homoeopathic Treatment

Sulphur 30C - Lesions are red and look wet; itching is intense, worse for warmth. Dose night and morning for 5 days.

Arsenic Alb 30C - If the hair falls off and the skin becomes loose and flabby or if there are ulcers with hard red edges, dry eczema, animal is thirsty and seeks warmth, symptoms worse after midnight, animal becomes more restless. This remedy is good to alternate with Sulphur. Dose once daily for 2 weeks.

Sepia 30C - If the effected parts are tender and the animal shrinks when touched or if there are white looking blisters filled with a watery fluid. Dose 3 times a day.

Rhus Tox 30C- Condition is vesicular and itchy, stiffness in joints which get better with movement. Dose 3 times daily.

Herbal Overview Of The Skin

Conditions such as wounds, burns, bites, ticks etc. are all dealt with in First Aid For Animals which gives detailed treatment for these conditions. For problems such as Ringworm look to the Anti-Fungal and Anti Biotic herbs, also consider lotions such as Calendula with Garlic and Tea Tree oil in a spray bottle so as to soak a area and for easy application. For the long drawn out chronic diseases of the skin use the Alteratives especially the ones with a strong affinity to the skin such as Sarsaparilla, Burdock, Cleavers and Nettles. The blood cleansers need time to do their work so always consider using them for 3 months as this is the life cycle of the red blood cells so you would of cleaned most of the blood after using them for this time.

Herbal Actions For The Skin

Alterative - Herbs that gradually restore proper function to the body, they increase health and vitality. They were once known as the blood cleansers.

Herbs - Black Cohosh, Blue Flag, Burdock, Cleavers, Chaparral, Echinacea, Fumitory, Garlic, Nettles, Pau D'Arco ,Sarsaparilla, Sweet Violets, Yellow Dock.

Anti-biotic - Echinacea, Garlic, Myrrh, Pau D' Arco, Tea Tree Oil

Anti-fungal - Marigold, Cats Claw, Pau D' Arco, Myrrh, Sweet Violets.

Anti-inflammatory - Helps the body to combat inflammations. Herbs mentioned under demulcents, emollients and vulneraries will often act in this way especially when they are applied externally.

Herbs - Arnica, Blue Flag, Cats Claw, Chaparral ,Chickweed, Cleavers, Cranesbill, Chamomile, Eyebright, Ginger, Golden Rod, Guaiacum, Licorice, Marshmallow, Marigold, Pau D' Arco, St John's Wort, Sweet Violets, Witch Hazel.

Astringent - Contracts tissue which in turn reduces discharges, these herbs contain tannins.

Herbs - Agrimony, Bear Berry, Cranesbill, Chaparral, Chickweed, Comfrey, Eyebright, Golden Rod, Hops, Horsetail, Ladys Mantle, Marigold, Marshmallow, Meadowsweet, Myrrh, Nettles, Raspberry, Sage, Rosemary, Slippery Elm, Shepherds Purse, St John's Wort, Slippery Elm, Thyme, Witch Hazel, Yarrow.

Emollient - Soothing to the skin. Acts externally the way demulcents do internally.

Herbs - Chickweed, Coltsfoot, Comfrey, Fenugreek, Licorice, Marshmallow, Mullein, Plantain, Slippery Elm.

Parasiticide - Kills parasites and insects.

Herbs - Aniseed, Rosemary,

Vulnerary - Applied externally and aid the body in the healing of wounds and cuts

Herbs - Arnica, Burdock, Chickweed, Comfrey, Cranesbill, Elder, Fenugreek, Garlic, Horsetail, Hyssop, Marigolds, Marshmallow,

Mullein, Myrrh, Plantain, Shepherds Purse, Slippery Elm, St John's Wort, Thyme, Witch Hazel, Yarrow.

Notes

The Reproductive System

Pregnancy

Consider worming after the sow becomes pregnant so as to lessen the burden on her and also to stop the young piglets from getting infested. Before the sow moves into the birthing area it is best to remove the old dung and clean the area thoroughly. Straw makes a good litter and bedding. Next do this to the pig, give her a good clean with soap and water, while doing this check for external parasites and any other potential problems then take her to the birthing area. Try to avoid any sudden changes in her diet try to keep it similar to what it was before. Fresh green feeds in small quantities may keep the sow interested in her food and is also laxative. Make sure the sow has easy access to water as this will be needed latter for a good milk supply.

Signs and Symptoms - Increased swelling and flabbiness of the vulva is a indication that birthing will begin soon and another good sign is milk appearing in the teats which usually means that there is about 12 hours to farrowing. At the onset of labor the birthing process usually takes 2 hours but always prepare for the worst. It is best to be there for the birth a good reason is that most piglets are born without their envelopes but if one comes out still in it the envelope must be removed or the piglet will suffocate. Usually the cord does not need much attention but can be wiped with a disinfectant. If the weather is cold the piglets will naturally seek the warmth of the mother's body and here you have to stop them from lying on top of other piglets and smothering them. Two signs of trouble are the sow straining for more than half an hour without effect and a delay of 2 hours without the next piglet arriving; you can tell if this is happening because the sow is ignoring the ones already born. In cases like this you may have to insert your fingers into the vagina and see if two piglets are trying to get out at the same time and blocking each other's path.

Warning - Sows are usually big animals and if you pick up a new born piglet and it squeals you may get attacked by a very upset sow. If you must pick one up grasp it by the mouth keeping its mouth shut so it cannot squeal while putting your other hand beneath its belly to lift it.

Herbal Treatment

Raspberry leaf is the most important herbal aid to a easy birth and should be given to all the breeders especially the ones that have difficult births. Herbs to think of to increase the milk are Marjoram, Sage, Fenugreek, Aniseed, Fennel and Speedwell.

Homoeopathic Treatment

Viburnum Opulis - A remedy for use in the early stages of pregnancy up to one month to 6 weeks. Helps to eliminate the tendency to early miscarriage. Give 30C three times per week for 4 weeks.

Caulophyllum - This remedy is used for the latter stages. Helps to ensure a trouble free birth and tones up the uterus for easy expulsion of the afterbirth. Give 30C three times per week for the last 4 weeks. If the last stage of labor is delayed or weak this remedy should be given again to help speed up normal contractions.

Arnica 30C - This can be used at the time of birthing and given for a few days after as it will help with the bruising and swelling and is good for shock. Give 3 times a day.

BellisPerennis 30C - If the birthing was prolonged or severe give this remedy along with Arnica.

Post Birth Problems

Retained Placenta

If you have a small amount of animals it is a good idea to have some sort of sick bay. I used to have a area for birthing and one of the most important reasons for this is that you would always know if the afterbirth had been expelled. In some cases parts of the afterbirth are expelled with the birth of the piglets but in most cases the afterbirth is passed with the birth of the last piglet usually within 3 to 5 hours. The first thing you should do after birthing is to get the piglets to suckle as this is the main trigger to release the after birth.

Herbal Treatment - Fast the Sow and then give a strong brew of raspberry leaf and linseed oil strengthened with honey or molasses. All of these substances are stimulating and tonic to the womb.

Feverfew can be added to the brew at one to one with the raspberry. Another herb to think of is Pennyroyal which is virtually the specific for this condition.

Homoeopathic Treatment

Homoeopathic remedies to consider are Sepia 30C, Pulsatilla 6c, Satilla 6C and Pyrogen 1M.

Sabina - Useful when the condition is associated with the retention of the afterbirth or miscarriage especially in those cases showing blood stained discharges. Give 6C every hour for 6 doses.

Hemorrhage

Herbal Treatment

Astringents are the main herbs that you use to stop bleeding. Two of the strongest ones are Shepherds Purse and Cranesbill. Make a 1 to 10 lotion of either of these herbs and if bleeding cannot be controlled use a small syringe without the needle to gently inject into the womb, hopefully this will spasm the ends of the bleeding vessels and stop the flow of blood. Give a strong dose internally as well.

Homoeopathic Treatment

Ipecacuanah 6C - Blood accumulates in the uterus and is then expelled in a bright red flood. Give every hour for 5 doses.

Crotalus 1M - If the blood comes away as a steady drip. Give every hour for 4 doses.

Hammamelis 30C - Dark blood indicating a venous origin will need this remedy. Give 1 dose every 2 hours up to 5 times.

Secale 30C - Very stringy blood indicates this remedy. Give 1 dose every 2 hours up to 5 times.

Metritis Acute

Metritis or inflammation of the womb can be acute or chronic. The acute condition is associated with the birth and is usually a bacterial invasion of the lining of the womb that comes within the first 3 days after birth. Chief among the causes of this condition is the retained placenta together with infection which gains entrance to the genital tract.

Symptoms - There is a rise in temperature, fever, followed by a loss of appetite and the sow is uneasy and lethargic. Respirations are increased and there may be a expression of anxiety on the face, abdominal pains, coma. The vulva and vagina may be inflamed and dark red. Discharge is not always present but if it is it may vary from a yellowish color through to blood stained and foul smelling.

Herbal Treatment

We will start off by telling you how this problem on the pregnancy side could have probably been avoided in the first place. If the sow was given the herbs Raspberry or Squaw Vine in the last months of pregnancy these herbs would have toned and strengthened the uterus and the problem may of been avoided. At the onset of labor if the herb Golden Seal was used it could have given the sow the extra strength and energy to have a successful and problem free labor, this usually works by making the contractions stronger. After the piglets are born it is usually when they start to suckle that triggers the expulsion of the placenta. Inflammations of the uterus arising from infection should be treated with the main immune boosting herbs mainly Echinacea, Garlic and another good one if you have got it is Myrrh. To these herbs consider adding Lady's Mantle (astringent) Black or Blue Cohosh, or Saw Palmetto. Cleavers could be used as a Alterative for cleaning out the system. A lotion of Calendula could be used to clean the outside area especially if it is red and sore also think of adding Hypericum to the lotion for pain relief.

Juliette de Bairacli Levy recommends an internal douche with a brew of lavender. If there was bleeding I would consider adding Lady's Mantle or shepherds purse to the douche. Calendula is another herb to think of adding.

Homoeopathic Treatment

Treatment should be started as bad signs start to appear after parturition especially after dead piglets and a difficult labor.

Aconitum 1M - Should be given at once so as to quickly allay shock, fear and anxiety and regulate the circulation. Give every hour for 4 hours.

Belladonna 1M - Indicated when the animal is hot to touch with a full bounding pulse and dilated pupils. Signs of cerebral excitement may be present with extreme cases convulsions. Give every hour for 5 hours.

Lillum Tig 30C - A good general remedy for uterine congestion leading to blood stained discharges and straining in the pelvic region.

Secale 30C- Hemorrhages are present when this remedy is considered, the blood is fluid and dark, the patient is cadaverous looking with cold extremities which are deficient in blood supply. Give twice daily for 10 days.

Sabina 6C- Useful when the condition is associated with the retention of the afterbirth or miscarriage especially in those cases showing blood stained discharges. Give every hour for 6 doses.

Pyrogen 1M - This nosode is indicated when a weak thready pulse alternates with a high temperature or vice versa. The most useful remedy in septic conditions. Give every 2 hours for 4 doses.

Mastitis

The cause can be a combination of factors such as faulty management, exposure to cold winds and wet weather, injuries from blows and sharp objects, and bacterial infections caught from others or as a result of poor hygiene. Mastitis can occur anytime during lactation but is frequently seen after birth.

Symptoms - Appetite fails and fever develops. Sometimes the temperature rises as high as 105 or 107 degrees. The entire udder rapidly hardens and becomes very hot to the touch. The affected glands are swollen, purple and may have a watery secretion. General signs include changes in milk secretion resulting in abnormalities such as clots and changes in the size and consistency of the udder parts involved. There is frequently also a systemic reaction. Sometime the sow tries to keep the legs from contacting the udder and as a result may walk with a different gait and stand with the rear legs apart. The acute form frequently comes after birth and a less severe form sometimes at drying off. The onset is usually sudden and can be recognized by swelling of the gland and changes in the milk. The swelling may take several forms ranging from slight edema to a hot painful enlargement. This condition can happen at any time during lactation. Isolate the effected sow and the piglets will have to be hand feed.

Herbal Treatment

The sow must be isolated and confined indoors for the treatment in a well-ventilated area. For the really stubborn cases begin with a cleansing fast of 2 days with water only allowed or water and a solution of molasses with a purge given in the evening. A effective purge is 2 ounces of Epsoms Salts, one ounce of linseed oil, half a teaspoonful of ground ginger, one teaspoonful of grated Gentian root and 2 ounces of warm water, give mixed in oatmeal gruel to make 1 and a half pints.   Garlic is the main herb to be given at the dosage of 1 whole root grated into one cup of water with half a cup given morning and night. Wood Sage (has a affinity to the udder) was also given with this treatment but is now very difficult to find.   Wood Sage can be made into a lotion and applied to the udder.

Humans sometimes use a cabbage leaf poultice for this condition, get some cabbage leafs and pound them so they are bruised all over and apply to the affected area, I will leave you to figure out how to do this as I aren't all that sure myself (adapted face mask?) as usually women use an oversized bra to hold the leaves in place. Photolacca tincture in small doses is the main herb for mastitis though I believe the Homoeopathic potency is far better and faster acting then the tincture.   To the Homoeopathic Dose you could make a lotion for external application of Photolacca but make it a very mild lotion as this is a strong remedy so make it about 1 to 20 in strength. The main immune boosting herbs should also be used these are Echinacea, Garlic and Myrrh as well as the alteratives such as Cleavers.

Homoeopathic Treatment.

A wise farmer would treat this on a herd basis by determining which bacteria is the cause and then making a Nosode (potency made from a disease product) of that bacteria to the 30C potency and treating the herd with it by dosing the animals water troughs.

Common frequent remedies used on a individual basis are as below.

Aconite 6X - This should be used as routine in all acute cases especially in those that develop suddenly, it will allay tension and restlessness, cause may be from exposure from cold dry winds. Dose every half hour for 6 doses.

Arnica 30C - Indicated when mastitis develops as a result of injury to the mammary tissue, blood may be present in the milk. Dose 3 times daily for 3 days.

Apis 6C - This is a useful remedy for freshly birthed sows showing edema of the udder and surrounding tissues. The mammary vein is usually engorged in this case. Dose every 3 hours for 4 doses.

Belladonna 1M - Indicated usually in the acute form post-partum. The udder shows acute swelling and redness, pain is obvious on touch, the animal will feel hot with full bounding pulse. Dose every hour for 4 doses.

Bryonia 30C - Indicated where the udder swelling is hard and indurated. In acute cases pain will be relieved by pressure on the udder and such cases are frequently presented with the animal lying down as this appears to give relief. Chronic forms showing fibrosis should benefit from this remedy. Dose 4 hourly for 4 doses while in the chronic form dose twice weekly for a month.

Phytolacca 30C - A useful remedy for both acute and chronic cases. Acute form may show curdled milk and clots while in the latter small clots may appear in mid lactation. This is probably the most useful remedy for the average chronic case. Dose 3 times daily for 3 days followed once daily for 4 days.

Urtica Urens 6X - For acute forms showing oedema which may be in the form of plaques frequently extending to the perineal area. Dose every hour for 4 doses.

Hepar Sulph 6X - This low potency will help promote suppuration and clearing of the udder contents in cases of C. Pyogenes or summer mastitis infection. Dose every 3 hours for 4 doses. Once the udder has been cleared of purulent material a dose or 2 of a higher potency should be given to complete the cure.

Ipecac 30C - This is a useful remedy for controlling intra-mammary bleeding which results in pink milk. Dose 3 times daily for 3 days.

Teats Sore or Damaged

The delicate tissues of the teat sometimes become chapped and develop deep fissures.

Symptoms - Damage or redness is seen and or the sow winces and will not tolerate the piglet from feeding.

Herbal Treatment - Juliette de Bairacli Levy recommends to treat alternately with warm almond oil as a salve and bathed with a brew of equal parts elder blossom and marshmallow. Raw cucumber juice has been effective. I would use Calendula and Hypericum Lotion (1 to 10) as this is a great healer of all wounds and also helps to relieve the pain.

Herbal Overview of The Reproductive System

Herbs to think of when a miscarriage is suspected are False Unicorn Root, Ladys Slipper, Blue Cohosh, Black Haw, Wild Yam, and Cramp Bark. The main herbs to think of for pregnancy are Raspberry, Squaw Vine and Shepherds Purse. Below are some of the actions to consider for this system. In the Astringents the herbs underlined are the best to use to stop bleeding. Use the Alteratives for Chronic diseases of this system and maybe add some of the Emmenagogues to them after reading up on the individual herbs and adding the one that works in the direction you want.

Herbal Actions For The Reproductive System

Alterative - Herbs that gradually restore proper function to the body, they increase health and vitality. They were once known as the blood cleansers.

Herbs - Black Cohosh, Dong Quai, Damiana, Skullcap.

Anti-biotic - Chaparral, Echinacea, Garlic, Myrrh, Pau D' Arco, Reshi.

Anti-fungal - Marigold, Cats Claw, Pau D' Arco, Myrrh, Sweet Violets.

Anti-inflammatory - Helps the body to combat inflammations. Herbs mentioned under demulcents, emollients and vulneraries will often act in this way especially when they are applied externally.

Herbs - Cranesbill, Chamomile, Eyebright, Feverfew, Ginger, Golden Rod, Lady's Mantle, Licorice, Marshmallow, Meadowsweet, Marigold, Pau D' Arco, St John's Wort, Witch Hazel.

Anti-Tumor - Burdock, Cleavers, Reshi, Shitake, Sweet Violets.

Antispasmodic - Prevents or eases spasms and cramps.

Herbs - Aniseed, Angelica, Black Cohosh, Chamomile, Fennel, Hyssop, Motherwort, Rosemary, Rue, Sage, Skullcap, St John's Wort, Thyme, Valerian, Vervain.

Anti-viral - Astragalus, Cats claw, Echinacea, Garlic, Myrrh?, Shitake, St John's Wort, Pau D'Arco.

Astringent - Contracts tissue which in turn reduces discharges, these herbs contain tannins.

Herbs - Agrimony, Cranesbill, Eyebright, Golden Rod, Ladys Mantle, Marigold, Raspberry, Shepherds Purse, St John's Wort, Witch Hazel.

Emmenagogue - Stimulates and normalizes the menstrual flow, tonics for the female reproductive system.

Herbs - Black Cohosh, Chamomile, Fenugreek, Gentian, Ginger, Juniper, Ladys Mantle, Marigold, Motherwort, Parsley, Penny Royal, Peppermint, Parsley, Raspberry, Sage, Rosemary, Rue, Shepherds Purse, St John's Wort, Tansy, Thyme, Valerian, Vervain, Wormwood, Yarrow.

Galactagogue - Helps increase the flow of milk in females.

Herbs - Aniseed, Fennel, Fenugreek, Milk Thistle, Raspberry, Vervain.

Infectious Diseases

Brucellosis

Caused by an organism named Brucella suis and occurs in most countries. Infection is spread by contact with infected stock especially from discharges from the alimentary and genital tracts. Piglets become infected by their mothers. Aborted fetuses and fetal membranes are a major source of spread. The disease is classed as venereal as sows are at risk from a infected boar. After exposure pigs develop bacteremia (bacteria in the blood) that may last for up to 90 days. During and after this localization may develop in various tissues with symptoms depending on which tissues are infected. Common symptoms may be abortion, sterility, orchitis, lameness, posterior paralysis, spondylitis and occasionally metritis and abscess formation in the extremities or other areas of the body. This disease can cross over to humans.

Symptoms - Abortion and infertility in sows, testicular swellings swelling of the lymph glands in the boar with posterior paralysis and lameness in both sexes, abortions can occur any time during pregnancy and are more common in those that have been infected by the boar.

Herbal Treatment

Start with our two main disease fighting herbs Garlic and Echinacea. Echinacea is good here for its action in fighting blood borne bacteria. The specific for this disease is Myrrh especially if there is lymphatic involvement. When the disease settles in the tissues look at the page that gives you the main herbs for that system. For this condition I would also consider large doses of Vitamin C and even injectable Vitamin C.

Homoeopathic Treatment

Give the nosode immediately to all stock as a prevention, isolate infected stock and also give these the nosode and consider the following remedies.

Hepar Sulph 30C - As this is a pyogenic infection this remedy may help especially with a sensitivity to cold and wind. Dose daily for 2 weeks.

Pyrogen 1M - This nosode is indicated when a weak thready pulse alternates with a high temperature or vice versa. The most useful remedy in septic conditions. Give every 2 hours for 4 doses.

Viburnum Opulis - A remedy for use in the early stages of pregnancy up to one month to 6 weeks. Helps to eliminate the tendency to early miscarriage. Give 30C three times per week for 4 weeks.

Caulophyllum - This remedy is used for the latter stages. Helps to ensure a trouble free birth and tones up the uterus for easy expulsion of the afterbirth. Give 30C three times per week for the last 4 weeks. If the last stage of labor is delayed or weak this remedy should be given again to help speed up normal contractions.

Leptospirosis

This disease may affect one or a group of animals with variable symptoms in each animal. There are two main species of leptospira the first being L. Pomona and the second being L. Icterohaemorrhagica . Infection is usually from urine of infected pigs or other wild life which enter the body via cuts and wounds or through moist surfaces such as the nose and mouth. After 3 to 5 days the infection is in the blood but persists in staying in two areas mainly the kidney and the reproductive tract. Abortions occurring 2 to 4 weeks before term are the most common symptoms in pigs. Piglets produced at term may be dead or weak and may die soon after birth.

Leptospirosis can be transmitted to human and can be fatal.

Symptoms - The disease requires moist environmental conditions to survive. Severe and mild forms of the disease are recognized. In the severe form the onset is sudden and comes after a short period of poor appetite and maybe fever. Signs of liver involvement appear with jaundice of the visible mucous membranes. Abortions are fairly constant. Milder forms show similar but less pronounced symptoms lasting only a few days. This is a very hard disease to diagnose.

Herbal Treatment

Give garlic and Echinacea. Echinacea is good here for its action in fighting blood borne bacteria. Refer to Jaundice if liver problems come on and also look at the Urinary System especially the urinary antiseptics.

Homoeopathic Treatment

Aconite 12X - Should be given as early as possible when the temperature is starting to rise. Dose every half hour for 4 doses.

Crotalus Horridus 200C - A very good remedy for controlling liver complications and reducing hemorrhages and jaundice. Dose every half hour for 4 doses.

Berberis 30C - Suitable for the milder case, will control liver dysfunction and may reduce haemoglobinuria. Dose 3 times daily for 2 days.

Phosphorus 1M - Another valuable liver remedy, will control the tendency to hemorrhages, faeces are generally clay colored. Dose once daily for 1 week.

Lycopodium 1M - Useful remedy for the convalescent stage when emaciation or loss of condition is apparent, will restore liver function and aid digestion. Dose daily for 1 week.

Refer to the remedies below to try and prevent abortions.

Viburnum Opulis - A remedy for use in the early stages of pregnancy up to one month to 6 weeks. Helps to eliminate the tendency to early miscarriage. Give 30C three times per week for 4 weeks.

Caulophyllum - This remedy is used for the latter stages. Helps to ensure a trouble free birth and tones up the uterus for easy expulsion of the afterbirth. Give 30C three times per week for the last 4 weeks. If the last stage of labor is delayed or weak this remedy should be given again to help speed up normal contractions.

Poisons

Acorns - Are a good food for pigs (not more the 10%of the ration) but an overdose may cause gastroenteritis and abortion in pregnant pigs. It is the shells that are dangerous due to their high tannic acid content. Normally the pigs split and discard the shells. The antidote is to give an oily purgative, 30 to 60ml of castor oil or flax seed oil depending on the size of the pig.

Bracken - When eaten this can destroy and prevent the absorption of vitamin B1. Sows and older pigs may develop a temperature, loose their appetite and even abort their piglets.

Buttercup - When grazing runs short in times of drought a sow may be forced to eat buttercup foliage. This can cause a soreness of the mouth developing into blisters and ulcers. Another effect of buttercup poisoning is diarrhea.

Castor Bean - Sometimes castor beans can get into the feed by mistake. Large seed contain a potent poison called ricin. Symptoms can be in a few hours and similar to botulism except that faeces often contain mucous and are often tinged with blood. Depression and paralysis are common. Pain due to inflammation of the bowel. Lethal dose can be as little as 2 large seeds. Poisoning is not as serious as it is in cattle because the pig is able to vomit. If poisoning is suspected encouraging vomiting by giving a emetic.

Cotton Seed - Contains gossypol which at certain levels can cause illness and death. Poisoning is slow to develop with evidence of muscular weakness, respiratory distress and generalized edema of the tissues especially the lung. The heart, liver and kidneys also show signs of degeneration and in some cases pin point hemorrhages.

Foxglove - Poisoning from eating foxglove is usually fatal. The active principle in this herb known as digitalis effects the heart and depending on the amount taken will cause excitement, quick respiration and heart beats, possibly followed by coma. Weaker heart beats then death.

Horsetail - This may cause scouring and loss of condition. Give an oily purgative, 30 to 60ml of castor oil or flax seed oil depending on the size of the pig.

Jute - The small gray seeds cause severe food rejection, vomiting and scouring in pigs.

Mexican Poppy - Small dark brown to black seeds like miniature peppercorns. The seed is extremely poisonous to humans and poultry. Seed at 2 to 6% in the feed of a 20kg pig causes severe food rejection by the second day. Symptoms of poisoning are lethargy, edema of the skin, lungs and lower limbs, reddening of the skin, oily yellow diarrhea and possibly hemorrhage.

Monkshood - Poisoning is usually fatal, death being due to asphyxia. In the early stages there may be salivation and staggering.

Nightshades - All three of the nightshades are poisonous to pigs. The poison affects the nerves and may lead to unconsciousness.

Potato Weed - Also called common Heliotrope. A annual weed infesting the wheat producing areas of South Australia. This weed causes liver damage. Low levels slowly damage the liver and severely effect growth without obvious signs.

Rhododendron - Are common in certain areas with acid soils. Symptoms may be salivation, vomiting, abdominal pain, depression of respiration, weakness, staggering gait and collapse.

Thorn apple - It is the seeds of this plant that can poison pigs when eaten. Symptoms can be gulpy swallowing, drunken movements, depression, dilated pupils, intense thirst, flushing of the skin, rapid pulse followed by coma and death.

Water Dropwort - This is a marsh loving plant whose roots are more dangerous to the pig then the foliage. Symptoms are diarrhea and maybe abdominal pains and convulsions. Give an oily purgative, 30 to 60ml of castor oil or flax seed oil depending on the size of the pig.

Notes

Herbal Supplement

Important Please Read

This Herbal Supplement is composed of herbs used for animals. We are going to concentrate on these Herbs as they are fairly safe. I have left in some of the dosages given to horses as a comparison. At the end of every section in the Cattle book for example The Digestive System there is an Overview of that section listing what are the common herbal actions needed for that system. The reason that is there is to teach you to think in the Actions you require for the treatment of your patient which gives you a more holistic view of the patient and what's happening. This makes you really start to think about what you are doing instead of thinking I will use the herb I used last time. Every case and every being is individual, think of what you are doing and why. Now for the hardest part, be patient, healing takes time. In the Actions explanation for example Demulcent, you will be told the meaning then given a list of herbs that are commonly known to be strong in that action, some will be different from what is listed in this herbal so you will have to do your own research but they should be generally safe for animal use as most of them come out of my Animal Herbal, this allows you a greater selection of herbs to use especially when you can't source the ones mentioned in the treatment section. Nearly all of the herbs mentioned have been historically used for animals and this is my part in making sure they are not forgotten again. I prefer using liquid to medicate in tinctures, extracts or infusion form even though there can be some controversy over the alcohol, the reason for this is that liquid spreads through the intestines a greater distance then the dry form which insures maximum absorption. In the herbal where no doses are mentioned these are the ones that are usually best in extract or tincture form and the manufacturers should give you the dose to match the strength that they have made it in.

Introduction to Herbal Medicine

Herbal Medicine has been in use and developed continuously since the beginning of time. It mainly evolved from observations from what plants did and the affects they had on people along with their animals. There is also what they call the Doctrine of Signatures which works like this, that flower really looks like an eye, maybe it helps sore eyes? I'll give it a try as my eyes are so sore and red. You know my eye really feels a lot better now, I think I will call that plant Eye Bright (Euphrasia) and tell my friends all about it especially my Dad who gets sore eyes to. In this way hundreds of plants were identified that have a medical action and no doubt there were also a lot of casualties.

The next great leap in herbal medicine was the Roman Empire of 2000 years ago. The Great Armies of Rome all had their own Medical Corps with Doctors, Battle Surgeons and Orderlies. It was these men who already had the knowledge of the Greeks that started to put together the best medical manuals in the world while at the same time started developing and using medical instruments and tools some of which are still used today. As the Romans conquered the known world more medicines and knowledge were found and assimilated.

The next great leap was modern Chemistry which allowed us to see exactly what herbs were made up of and what parts of the herb causes its medical action. Drug companies have made billions of Dollars from this information as they find the main active ingredient and then make a synthetic version of it, one good example that we all know of is Valium which is the synthetic version of the active ingredient from the herb Valerian. Leaving aside the Drug Companies let's see how Chemistry changed the way that modern herbalists think.

Modern science allows us to now know what Actions our herbs perform on the body so we shall carry on using Valerian as a example and see what Medical Actions Valerian has on the body.

The Actions of Valerian are Sedative, Hypnotic (sleep inducing), Anti Spasmodic (stops twitches, cramps etc), Hypotensive (lowers Blood Pressure) and Carminative (calms and relaxes the tummy). Herbalists call Valerian the Herbal Tranquillizer and if you look at the above you can see why for if you can't sleep and your blood pressures up along with a gurgling tummy and a eye constantly twitching you definitely need to be calmed down.

The modern herbalist is trained to think in actions. There are many reasons for this but the main ones are to stop them from just using a handful of their favorite herbs and to train the mind to work in the method of thinking in actions that are needed. If we start thinking in the actions that are needed for a patient it makes us consider the problem in far more depth than just using our favorite herb and it forces our thinking to be far more holistic by taking in consideration the whole of the patient not just the part or the system we wish to treat.

Let's take a look at thinking in actions. The animal has a cough, but when it coughs it can't stop and the cough sounds a bit like whooping cough. The animal also sounds a little hoarse and the temperature is also elevated. The actions that come into mind for this are expectorant for the cough, anti spasmodics for the whooping quality of the cough and demulcents to sooth the sore throat. These are the obvious actions and we can add many more if we wish such as immune boosters for acute diseases, diaphoretics to reduce the temperature and prevent a fever and the list goes on. Next we look at how Herbal Actions are used in making Herbal Formulas.

Another point to make before we go to the formula making is that Professional Herbalists use Herbs in the form of Tinctures (water and alcohol solutions) as this allows them to mix formulas in any proportions that they like and also allows long term storage without spoiling.

Making Herbal Formulas

You should never have more the 5 Herbs in a herbal formula otherwise you start to lose track of what you are doing and how the formula is changing the symptoms. Always try to keep things simple. One of the herbs in the formula is used to force the formula into the body, to keep it simple we will only use three, they are Licorice, Ginger and Cayenne.

As an example let's use an animal with a cough. After further study of the case we decide that this is a Acute Disease for it came on quick and is fast acting not slow like a Chronic Disease. Listening to the animals cough we decide that it is a dry cough and upon looking at the animal's nose we can't see any mucus. Let's list the actions to consider.

Expectorants - Licorice, Aniseed, Fennel, Garlic and Mullein

Antispasmodics - Aniseed and Fennel

Demulcents - Licorice and Coltsfoot

Immune Boosters - Echinacea

Anti-Bacterial and Virals - Garlic and Echinacea

Out of the above I would choose Licorice, Echinacea, Garlic, Aniseed and Fennel. I would make the formula in this strength.

Formula

Licorice - 20%

Garlic - 15%

Echinacea - 15%

Aniseed - 30%

Fennel - 20%

Look these herbs up in the herbal and consider why I used them, there are three obvious ones for Licorice alone with the first being to force the assimilation of the formula into the body, second is its expectorant action and third is its demulcent action in case the throat is sore and raw. Next time you see a little kid eating heaps of licorice get them to open their mouth and look at their tongue which will be going black from the Licorice along with the throat etc and know that you are looking at the demulcent action of Licorice working by coating and soothing.

The most important reason that you use the Actions Method for Herbal Prescribing is so that you can concentrate the Actions which are most needed for example, if it's a Bacterial infection concentrate on the Anti Bacterials, if it's a Viral infection concentrate on the Anti Virals, hopefully you are now beginning to see the importance of working in actions for if you don't concentrate a large part of the battle on the causes you may have lost the battle from the start.

Read through all the Actions listed in Herbal Actions at the end of each body system in the book and then do a study in depth of at least five Actions of your choice making the first two the Anti Bacterials and Anti Virals. Start trying to train your mind into thinking in Actions.

How to Make Herbal Tinctures

Tinctures are made by steeping the Herb plant material in a mixture of alcohol and water. Alcohol is usually always used at a strength of 45%. The alcohol in this mixture will extract all the essential oils from the herb while the water will extract all that is water soluble, so between the both we are getting most of the medicinal properties out of the herb.

The proportions of herb to liquid are usually 1 part herb to 5 parts liquid. So find a suitable container (I use a big one liter preserving jar with a good sealing lid) and put into it 100grams of your chosen herb and to that add 500mls of our 45% solution of alcohol. Seal the lid and shake well for about a minute. Leave the jar on the window sill so the sun can shine on the jar for two weeks. The jar must be shaken for at least a minute every day.

After 2 weeks open and filter the contents of the jar. I use a large pouring jug into which I place a funnel and then place a coffee filter in the funnel and pour the jar contents through the funnel being careful not to let too much herb spill into the filter and block it up. When you get to the bottom of the jar you can crush the herb in your fist so as to extract the last of the liquid.

After this is completed you then get your chosen storage bottle, put a funnel into its neck followed by a coffee filter and then filter the jug into the bottle. Remember the solution should always be double filtered

Next we label the bottle, put the date, name and proportions eg 1 to 5 also state the recommended dose. Store in a cool and dark place. Most Professional Homoeopaths and Herbalists have access to pure alcohol so for them it is fairly easy to make tinctures while for the lay person they will probably have a hard time. An alternative is to use Vodka as strong as you can find it or find a way to twist the authorities arm into giving alcohol at 45%. Don't even try to get pure alcohol as it is dangerous and can turn people blind and they won't give it to you.

How to Make Infusions

Infusions are a bit like making a cup of tea except we don't use milk. Infusions are used for the soft parts of the herb such as the flowers, leaves and fine twigs. The proportions for infusions are 1 to 20 eg 1 part herb to 20 parts water. Infusions are used for the more water soluble herbs.

Infusions can be made from a single herb or from a combination of herbs and may be drunk hot or cold. The water should be just off the boil before being poured on the herb and if you are making a infusion of a herb strong in essential oils such as Peppermint always cover the top of the cup to stop the essential oils from escaping in steam while the infusion is brewing. Allow up to 10 minutes to brew. It is best to make herbal teas fresh each day. You can experiment on yourself by getting Chamomile and Peppermint tea bags from the supermarket. Use honey as a sweetener.

How to Make Decoctions

Decoctions are used for the more hard woody substances of the herb such as barks, berries or roots. The process of decoction is far more vigorous then infusion as it involves heating the plant material in cold water, bringing it to the boil and simmering for 20 to 40 minutes. The finished ratio for decoctions is again 1 part herb to 20 parts water, remember to add more water at the beginning so you wind up with the 1 to 20 after steam loss. This form of preparation is no good for the herbs that are high in essential oils as these will all be lost in the steam.

How to Make Poultices

Poultices are used to sooth, irritate or draw impurities from the skin so choose your required plants by the actions you need. A Poultice is used to apply a remedy to the skin with moist heat and slight pressure. To prepare a poultice bruise or crush the fresh medicinal parts of the herb you are using into a pulpy mass and add a little hot water if needed. If using dried herb moisten the material by mixing with a hot soft adhesive substance such as moist flower and cornmeal or as they did in the past a mixture of bread and milk. This can be done to the fresh herb if you want as well. For ease of application to the skin it is best to spread the mixture on cheese cloth and fold to the appropriate size or shape required. The cloth also helps by retaining the moisture and even allows you to tie it gently the affected area. Moisten the cloth with hot water periodically when and if needed. Hot water bottles can also be used to keep the poultice warm. Always keep some cloth between the skin when using irritant plants such as mustard and always wash the skin thoroughly after use.

Dosage For Forms Of Herbal Medicines

Herbs can be given to animals in several different forms depending on what best suites the herb, the ailment, and the condition of the animal and of what is available at the time and then most importantly the expense.

Herbal Extract - Are alcohol based and about the strongest herbal preparation you can get as they nearly extract everything from the herb. Generally the strength is every ml should be equivalent to one gram of the herb. Used and dosed the same as tinctures but the dose will always be less than what is used in a tincture. From this try to work out if the extra price is worth it. Supplier should give dosage.

Tincture - Is a weaker then Herbal Extracts but also made from alcohol. Dilute the appropriate number of drops in water for treatment. Supplier should give dosage.

Infusion - A infusion is like making a cup of tea out of the flowers and leaves and other soft parts of the herb. Add boiling water and cover so as all the essential oils don't escape in the steam and leave for 20 minutes.

Decoction - Usually made from the root, bark or seed and is simmered for a while to extract the medicinal properties. Usually dosed the same as infusions.

Powdered - These are usually made from roots and bark and given in doses from a teaspoon to tablespoon. These can also be infused and turned into a tea. Try to get powdered extracts as they are more the real thing instead of for example powdered Ginger at the supermarket.

Fresh Herb - This is the easiest way to medicate a horse just add a large handful of the leaves to the feed. Always check for woody parts and sharp stalks. For dangerous or strong herbs chop finely and mix thoroughly into moistened feed so no one animal eats too much.

Dried Herb - Most dried herb is usually cut, again run your hand through for wood or sharps. If you are growing the herb yourself cut up or grind and mix directly with the feed. Crushed herbs can also be mixed with water and formed into a pill for individual treatment or the whole stable can be dosed in a mix with feed.

Note - Always be guided by the recommended dose of the individual herb instead of working in generals.

Calculating Correct Herbal Doses for Animals

Cats - 1/8 to 1/6 the dose for an adult human.

Dogs - Correspond to adult human dose according to weight.

Horse - 8 to 16 times the dose for an adult human.

Goats - 2 times the dose for an adult human.

Sheep - 1 1/2 times the dose for an adult human.

Cow - 12 to 24 times the dose for an adult human.

Swine - 1 to 3 times the dose for an adult human.

Not all herbs are of the same strength so for this reason it is a good idea to always look at the human dose and if this dose seems to be lower than normal, do your research into why. It might be a good idea to have a look at the herb Poke Root just to see what a strong herb looks like and can do.

Animal Herbal

Agrimony

Actions - Astringent, tonic, diuretic, vulnerary, cholagogue.

Used as a remedy for jaundice, it should be given to fasting animal as a drench or finely cut and mixed with bran, it is also a valuable astringent to stem bleeding and is a remedy for sore throats. Sprains are aided by a lotion made by boiling one handful of chopped Agrimony in one quart of brew made from wheaten bran. The combination of astringency and of bitter tonic properties make this a powerful herb for the digestive system. This is a good and gentle remedy for the young.

Uses - Diarrhea in the young, mucous colitis, spring tonic, indigestion, urinary incontinence and cystitis, as a gargle for sore throats and laryngitis and as a ointment or lotion for wounds and bruises.

Cautions - Not to be used during Pregnancy

Alfalfa

Rich in nitrates and vitamins is a good tonic food and a kidney cleanser. Excellent for all animals and poultry. Fodder, tonic, nervine, aids in healing allergies, arthritis, morning sickness, peptic ulcers, stomach ailments and bad breath, removes poisons from the body, neutralizes acids, is a excellent blood purifier and thinner, improves appetite and aids in the assimilation of protein, calcium and other nutrients.

Angelica

Actions - Expectorant, anti-spasmodic, diaphoretic, diuretic, carminative.

Useful expectorant for coughs, bronchitis and pleurisy especially when they are accompanied by fever, colds or influenza. The leaf can be used as a compress in inflammations of the chest. Its high oil content helps in intestinal colic and flatulence. Can ease rheumatic inflammations, in cystitis it acts as a urinary antiseptic.

Uses - Coughs, bronchitis, pleurisy, colic, wind, rheumatic inflammations, cystitis.

Aniseed

Actions - Expectorant, antispasmodic, carminative, parasiticide, aromatic.

Dogs like aniseed so much that it was once used as a bait by dog thieves. As a carminative it is unsurpassed. A important remedy for all digestive ailments including colic.

Uses - Gripping, intestinal colic, wind, as a expectorant in bronchitis, tracheitis, irritable coughing, whooping cough

External - The oil by itself will help in the control of lice and scabies.

Dose - Average dose for horses is one handful of seeds daily.

Arnica

Actions - Anti-inflammatory, vulnerary.

For external use only Homoeopathic preparations can be used internally. For the treatment of shock and pains from accidents, bruises, joint stiffness and wounds, swellings, paralysis, sprains, rheumatic conditions or where ever there is inflammation on the skin.

Caution - Do not apply to open wounds or broken skin.

Homoeopathy - Used from 3C to 200C orally for injury, bleeding, bruising, shock or for any conditions that feel bruised or have a bruised like feeling.

Astragalus

Actions - Immune-modulator, anti-viral, adaptogen, hypotensive, immune stimulant, adrenal tonic, diuretic, circulatory stimulant, vasodilator, blood tonic.

This herb should only be used in chronic diseases, as a preventative or in cases of fatigue especially in chronic diseases. Stimulates the natural production of interferon and intensifies the white cell destruction of germs.

A good tonic for strengthening the resistance to disease. Is very useful for animals in a state of chronic debility and fatigue by restoring the immune function. Use as a lung tonic to help expel toxins and pus in flu's, colds and sinusitis. Increases stamina and can accelerate wound healing, can help to replenish bone marrow. Strengthens the digestive system and aids adrenal gland function. This herb is used for cancer especially if the patient has had chemotherapy and helps aid them in their recovery.

Uses - Boosting immune system, disease preventative, fatigue, healing wounds. This is a good herb to use before and during a long distance or time consuming transportation.

Cautions - Should not be used in acute infections or fevers.

Barberry

Actions - Cholagogue, anti-emetic, bitter tonic, laxative, alterative, hypotensive, and antibacterial.

Good for correcting liver function and increasing the flow of bile. The herb is also a bitter tonic and mild laxative, use for weak and debilitated animals to strengthen and clean the system. Has been known to reduce enlarged spleens and also act against malaria. Its antibacterial properties have shown activity against strep, staph salmonella, shigella and eschorichia. This herb also dilates blood vessels thus lowering blood vessels.

Uses - Inflammation of the gallbladder, stones, liver problems, jaundice, arthritis, intestinal infections.

Cautions - Use only the dried plant and avoid during pregnancy.

Bear Berry - Uva Ursi

Actions - Diuretic, astringent, antiseptic and demulcent.

Bear Berry has a specific antiseptic and astringent effect on the membranes of the urinary system and will generally soothe tone and strengthen them. It is specifically used where there is gravel or ulceration in the kidneys or bladder. A very useful herb where there is cystitis.

Uses - Urinary infections, gravel and ulcerations in the urinary system also to soothe these areas.

Black Cohosh

Actions - Emmenagogue, anti-spasmodic, alterative, sedative.

Has hormone balancing properties, encourages oestrogen production, good for pets that loose hair after being spayed, painful or delayed menstruation, ovarian cramps, cramping pain, used to regain normal hormone activity, rheumatoid and osteoarthritis, muscular and neuralgic pains.

Blue Flag

Actions - Cholagogue, alterative, laxative, diuretic, anti-inflammatory.

Often called liver lily which shows its use in liver ailments. It acts as a general conditioner for the whole system and is also a gentle laxative. Stimulates the digestive glands. This is usually used with other blood cleansers and should be used in small doses at first in case it stirs up to much rubbish.

Uses - Treatment of all liver ailments, jaundice, gall bladder disorders, general tonic, appetizer, mild laxative, eczema, skin diseases, psoriasis.

Boswella

Actions - Anti-inflammatory, anti-arthritic, astringent.

Good for use in any of the chronic inflammations in any body system.

Uses - Lung diseases especially of the chronic kind with inflammation, rheumatic diseases, diarrhea, dysentery, piles, STDs. It is also used in general weakness.

Broom

Actions - Cardioactive diuretic, hypertensive, peripheral vasoconstrictor, astringent.

Russian peasants use Broom tops as a very successful remedy for rabies. It is also used as a mild vermifuge. The flowers infused in hot milk (one handful to one pint) are used internally and externally to cure severe forms of skin ailments. The young twigs are mildly purgative.

Uses - Worms, skin ailments, rabies, dropsy, constipation, increases flow of urine in kidney ailments, used where there is a weak heart and low blood pressure, profuse menstruation.

Caution - Do not use in pregnancy and high blood pressure.

Burdock

Actions - Alterative, diuretic, bitter, antibacterial, anti-tumor.

It is used to treat conditions arising from an "overabundance" of toxins, such as boils, rashes and chronic skin problems. Helps to cleanse the body of waste products. Animals will not graze this herb with the exception of the ass, but the sliced and bruised roots are one of the finest blood cleansers known to herbalists. The bruised leaves applied externally are a remedy for ring worm and scabies. Soothing to the kidneys and a excellent diuretic. The juice is used internally for scabies and mites.

Uses - Remedy for all blood disorders, rheumatism, skin parasites , skin conditions resulting in dry scaly skin, psoriasis, eczema, dandruff, aids digestion and appetite, aids kidney function and helps with cystitis, speeds up the healing of wounds and ulcers. Use to reduce tumors.

Buchu

Actions - Diuretic, urinary antiseptic, digestive tonic, kidney tonic.

Used in any infection of the genito-urinary system such as cystitis, urethritis and prostatitis. Especially useful in painful and burning urination. Good kidney tonic. Used to treat blood in the urine, stones and chronic urinary infections especially if started by colon bacteria.

Cayenne

Actions - Stimulant, carminative, tonic, sialagogue, rubefacient, anti-septic.

Used as a catalyst to help push herbal formulas into the body. Aids heart failure (a few drops on the side of the mouth), stimulates the heart, helps heal ulcers of the stomach and colon, cayenne powder sprinkled on a open wound stops bleeding, flatulent dyspepsia, colic. Externally it is used as a rubefacient in problems like lumbago and rheumatic pains.

Caution - High doses on an empty stomach can cause gut irritation and eventually ulcers

Calendula

Actions - Anti-inflammatory, astringent, vulnerary, anti-fungal, cholagogue, emmenagogue.

Goats and sheep seek it out, the flowers are tonic and a good heart medicine they possess restorative powers over the arteries and veins, the flowers are also fed to make miserable fretting animals cheerful, also used for liver problems, vomiting, internal ulcers.

Uses - Cuts, grazes, infected sores, fungal infections, any skin inflammations, regulates the oil production of the skin so is good for acne, to stop bleeding, bruises and sprains, skin ulcers and minor burns and scolds, healing, soothing, anti-microbial. Use as a lotion to clean wounds, one of our main germicides for wounds and if Hypericum is added to the lotion you may prevent tetanus as well.

Use externally as a lotion (1 to 20) or a cream.

Caution - Calendula closes wounds rapidly so make sure they are very clean and no foreign bodies remain.

Cat Mint

Actions - Carminative, antispasmodic, diaphoretic, sedative, astringent.

This herb is also known as Catnip. Cats and other creatures eat this plant and also give themselves a massage in it. This plant sometimes causes cats to grow pensive and dreamy. This is an old traditional cold and flu remedies especially ones with fever. Has a action on the digestive system easing stomach upsets, dyspepsia, wind and colic. Used for diarrhea of the young. Good for nervous, stressed or restless animals.

Cats Claw

Actions - Anti oxidant, immune stimulant, anti-inflammatory, anti-fungal, anti-rheumatic, anti-viral, anti-tumor, anti-microbial.

To alleviate allergic sinus type conditions, boost the immune system, asthma, bursitis, Candida, immune deficiency disorders, chronic inflammatory diseases, auto immune conditions.

Cautions - Don't use during pregnancy.

Celery Seed

Actions - Anti rheumatic, diuretic, carminative, sedative, alterative, hypotensive.

The main use for this herb is in the treatment of rheumatism, arthritis and gout. Celery seed can help soothe the nerves and relieve pain and also aids the body in the removal of uric acid. A good cleansing, mildly diuretic herb, useful in ridding the system of an accumulation of waste products. An improvement in circulation of fluids encourages a horse to drink and sweat more easily. Celery seed mixed with food aids in the digestion of protein. A very good digestive tonic if the horse is run down with little appetite.

Uses - Arthritis, hyperacidity, pain, hypertension, digestion, urinary tract infections

Centaury

Actions - Bitter, aromatic, mild nervine, gastric stimulant, chologogue, febrifuge, vermafuge.

Use whenever a gastric stimulant is required especially in cases of anorexia and liver weakness. This is a good herb for use in the young.

Uses - For digestive ailments, jaundice, as a vermafuge including liver fluke, use externally for lice, wounds and warts. In the past it was also used as a birth remedy.

Chamomile

Actions - Carminative, sedative, anti-spasmodic, anti-inflammatory, analgesic and anti-septic.

It is a famed blood cleanser and pain reducer, reduces tumors (poultice), remedy for female ailments, inflamed gums, use for blood and skin disorders, aches and pains, external and internal inflammations, delayed menstruation, acid uterus and all female ailments, cleanser and toner of the digestive tract, it is well documented as having anti-inflammatory activity and is also beneficial in reducing allergic responses as it contains a number of anti-histamine chemicals. In addition, it is recognized as being ulcer-protective through its healing effect on the mucosa of the gastro-intestinal tract, expels worms and parasites, improves and helps appetite. Good for nervous and hyperactive horses as it calms them without making them tired.

Uses - Indigestion, colic, diarrhea, teething, anxiety, insomnia, nervous upsets, slowing down hyperactive horses, flatulence. Good all round tonic for the nervous system especially for nervous animals.

Chaparral

Actions - Alterative, astringent, diuretic, tonic, powerful antioxidant, anti-arthritic, anti-rheumatic, anti-cancer, anti-tumor, dissolves calculi, anti-biotic.

Uses - Used in kidney problems and stones and for rheumatism and arthritis. Aids in healing skin blemishes, acne, allergies, promotes hair growth, acts as a natural anti-biotic, cataracts, has a action on cancer.

Chaste Tree

Actions - Emmenagogue, galactagogue, Tonic for the reproductive organs.

More of a hormone balancer by working directly on the pituitary gland though is more of a normalizing herb, usually increases the progesterone levels therefore increasing the chance of pregnancy. Supporting the progesterone level is extremely helpful in counteracting the irritability and unpredictability that can happen with mares in season making them more comfortable, cooperative and safer to handle. Though this herb is primarily used to balance hormonal irregularities in mares it can also be used to inhibit the sex hormones of stallions if their behavior is thought dangerous or seen to be causing them a loss in condition. Useful on its own or in combination with herbs specific for hormonal balance.

Used for endometriosis, fibroids, infertility and threatened miscarriages.

Chickweed

Actions - Healing, anti-inflammatory, astringent, emollient.

Rich in copper, highly tonic food for the digestive system and a remedy for all stomach ailments, allergies, colon problems, constipation, piles, rheumatism, skin problems, eczema, psoriasis, itching, irritation, cuts and wounds.

Uses - One of the main uses of this herb is for itching skin conditions whether from insect bites or eczema like conditions. Has wound healing and demulcent properties.

Cleavers

Actions - Alterative, diuretic, anti-inflammatory, astringent, tonic, anti-cancer.

A lymphatic tonic with alterative and diuretic actions which can be used in a wide range of problems where the lymphatic system is involved. The plant is very rich in minerals and silica, gives good strong texture to the hair of animals and strengthens the hoofs. Also used to ease swollen legs and joints, support the lymphatic and endocrine systems and encourage the elimination of toxins, is also helpful if your horse experiences muscle tightening during or after exercise. All animals eat it and poultry especially seek it hence its popular name of goose grass. Good for skin ailments.

Uses - Tonic, eczema, abscesses and tumors, cancerous growths, swollen glands, tonsillitis, psoriasis, cystitis.

Coltsfoot

Actions - Expectorant, anti-tussive, demulcent, anti-catarrhal, diuretic.

The Latin name means banish cough. Coltsfoot combines a soothing expectorant action with a anti-spasmodic action. There are useful zinc levels in this plant. Consider this herb in any respiratory problem.

Uses - Coughs, pneumonia, asthma, pleurisy, TB, sedative powers in epilepsy, chronic or acute bronchitis, emphysema, cystitis.

Externally - A poultice is used for abscess, ulcers, boils, earache and toothache.

Comfrey

Actions - Demulcent, astringent, healing, expectorant.

Once widely cultivated as a fodder plant, sheep and cows eat it greedily, the impressive wound healing powers of comfrey are partially due to allantoin which stimulates cell proliferation and speeds the healing process inside and out. Has been used for thousands of years as a herb with abilities to mend broken bones. Has the same result on wounds, tendons, fractures, sprains, ulcers and cartilage.

Uses - Its old name is knit bone and that describes well what it does. Comfrey also guards against scar tissue from developing incorrectly, all internal hemorrhages including uterine, reunion of wound and fractures, internal ulcers, ruptures, pulmonary problems, bronchitis, irritable cough, ulcerative colitis, skin ulcers and varicose veins.

Corn Silk

Actions - Diuretic, demulcent, tonic, antiseptic, antilithic.

A soothing diuretic that is helpful in any irritation of the membranes of the urinary system. Combined with other herbs in the treatment of cystitis, urethritis and prostatitis. Cleanses and soothes the urinary system.

Cranesbill

Action - Strong astringent, anti-inflammatory, vulnerary.

One of the best astringents known for internal and external use and is palatable to most animals.

Uses - Dysentery and diarrhea especially in the old and young, piles, duodenal or gastric ulcers, uterine hemorrhage or any internal bleeding especially of the digestive and respiratory systems, douche in leucorrhoea, treatment of wounds.

Cranberry

Actions - Urinary antiseptic

Cranberry inhibits the adhesion of bacteria to the urinary pipe lines so each time water is passed the bacteria is flushed out thus preventing recolonization.

Dandelion

Actions - Diuretic, cholagogue, anti-rheumatic, laxative, tonic

The leaves of the Dandelion plant are generally fed to horses during spring as the herb assists with cleansing the blood. They are high in iron and calcium as well as Vitamins A, B, and D and are traditionally used as a tonic to stimulate the bladder.

The herb is blood cleansing and tonic, it has a important effect on the hepatic system and is a supreme jaundice curative herb, the leaves strengthen the enamel of the teeth and the white   juices of the freshly crushed stem dissolves warts, the plant is well grazed by goats, horses will take quantities of the leaves when cut and well mixed with bran. Dandelion Root is helpful for horses recovering from an illness or a reaction to vaccination. Being a tonic, this herb assists to clean the liver, kidneys and blood and is high in potassium and magnesium. Excellent for anemia because it is high in iron, calcium, copper and vitamins, useful in kidney and bladder problems, skin eruptions, sluggish blood flow, weak arteries, all liver complaints, jaundice, constipation, gallbladder problems and rheumatism.

Devils Claw

Actions - Anti-inflammatory, pain killer, hepatic, anti-rheumatic, alterative.

Used for its analgesic and anti-inflammatory properties, it is useful for treating pain in a range of joint and muscular problems. The bitter action of Devils Claw stimulates and tones the digestive system. Good for reducing inflammation in arthritis, gout and rheumatism. Aids the body in the elimination of uric acid. This plant also aids liver and gallbladder complaints.

Caution- Use with demulcent herbs to save irritating the tummy, don't use on horses with ulcers.

Dong Quai

Actions - Emmenagogue, antispasmodic, analgesic, uterine tonic ,vasodilator, hormone balancer, alterative.

Known regulator for the female reproductive system. Some of its compounds stimulate the uterus while others relax the uterus. The compounds that stimulate the uterus are water soluble and are absorbed into the body from teas and capsules. The compounds that relax the uterus are soluble in alcohol and are provided by tinctures. This herb may stop cramping, and ease the pain of ovarian cysts. The Chinese use this herb for abnormal menstruation, suppressed flow, painful or difficult menstruation. This herb is also good for the treatment of psoriasis. Dong Quai also helps with , asthma, bronchitis, emphysema and improves the function of the lungs. Builds and improves circulation as well as disperses congestion in the pelvic area.

Cautions - Avoid during pregnancy and in cases with diarrhea and dysentery.

Echinacea

Actions - Immune stimulant, anti-microbial, anti-inflammatory, alterative, healing.

Is a infection fighter active against strep bacteria (abscesses and boils), a blood cleanser, (blood poisons, snake bites, poisonous insects) and a glandular and lymphatic system cleanser. Use it particularly for respiration infections and for any disease above the waist. This is one of our main immune boosters for the acute diseases. Use as a prophylactic to protect horses from infections especially when traveling.

Uses - All infections, depressed immune function, inflammatory conditions, allergies, effective against both bacteria and viruses.

Warning - Do not use continually as you will burn out the immune system give a few weeks break after 3 weeks. Beware also in the use of allergies for you could be building up the immune system just to attack itself.

Elecampane

Actions - Expectorant, antitussive, anti-bacterial, antifungal, diaphoretic, stomachic, demulcent.

This herb is meant to be named after Helen of Troy and is a very ancient herb used for thousands of years especially by the Romans. Specific for irritating bronchial coughs, lots of catarrh, has a soothing and anti-bacterial action.

Mainly used for treating chronic coughs, bronchitis and asthma especially in the young. . It is also used for digestive problems. Elecampane also contains Alantolactone which helps to expel intestinal parasites such as pin worm. A external wash can help deter Scabies.

Uses - Bronchitis, emphysema, asthma and digestive problems. In the past was used for TB.

Elder

Actions - Diaphoretic, diuretic, anti-catarrhal, expectorant.

Most animals will graze on elder. Used for the treatment of all gastric, hepatic, and pulmonary ailments, all fevers, skin disorders especially scabies and ring worm, externally as a insecticide.

Leaves - Externally emollient and vulnerary (bruises, sprains and wounds). Internally used as a purgative, expectorant, diuretic and Diaphoretic. Topically the lotion makes a anti-inflammatory wash, salve, eyewash and gargle for sore throats.

Flowers - Diaphoretic and Anti catarrhal. Use for colds and flu.

Berries - Diaphoretic and Anti catarrhal. The uses are similar to the flowers but the berries are used for rheumatism. The berries have been used as a nutrient rich tonic given after birth to help build the blood.

Eye Bright

Actions - Anti-inflammatory, astringent, anti-catarrhal.

As the name says this is one of the main herbs in the treatment of eye problems. The aerial (above ground) parts of the plant are used. As its name suggests, it helps eye problems by relieving inflammation and tightening mucous membranes and is specifically used in treating conjunctivitis and blepharitis. Used for infections and allergic conditions affecting the eyes, middle ear, sinuses and nasal passages.

The plant is also nervine, tonic and astringent. Its use is both internal and external strengthening greatly the eyes nerves when used so. The high potassium and sulphur content of the plant make it also of value in treatment of gastric ailments especially insufficiency of gastric juices. Acts as a internal medicine for the constitutional tendency to eye weakness.

Uses- Best known for its use in the eye where it is helpful in acute or chronic inflammations, stinging and weeping eyes, over sensitivity to light, conjunctivitis, allergies, sinusitis, ulcers and general eye weakness.

Fennel

Actions - Carminative, aromatic, anti-spasmodic, stimulant, galactagogue, expectorant.

The herb possesses highly antiseptic and tonic properties. The primary use of fennel is to relieve bloating, but it also settles stomach pain, stimulates the appetite and is diuretic and anti-inflammatory. Peasants drive their flocks to feed upon it owing to the abundance of milk that the herb produces and the sweet odor that it imparts upon the milk. (if the animal is not native they can over gorge and poison themselves).

Arabs use fennel poultices to resolve old and hard tumors.

Uses - Gastric ailments, relieves flatulence and colic, stimulates appetite, inflammation of the bowels, acute constipation (raw roots daily), fevers, cramps, worms, indigestion, all eye ailments, bronchitis, coughs, muscular and rheumatic pains use the oil. Externally used as a eye wash to treat eye infections.

Fenugreek

Actions - Expectorant, demulcent, tonic, carminative, galactagogue, alterative, restorative.

Strongly aromatic herb, and the seeds of the plant are used. It contains a volatile oil, flavonoids, mucilage, protein, Vitamins A, B & C, alkaloids, saponins and some minerals. The seeds can aid in recovery from illness and to encourage weight gain. This is a herb well worth getting to know not just because of its tonic properties but for its rubbish removing actions especially in mucous thick chronic diseases such as sinusitis. Always use cleansing herbs like this one slowly and at a low doses especially when using for long periods of time. The plant possesses highly aromatic seeds having a powerful disinfectant, emollient and lubricant properties. The feeding value of these is about equal to linseed. It is one of the great fattening herbs. The perfect sister herb for garlic enhancing all its powers. Very tonic and eagerly sought by all animals. Rich in vitamins and nitrates, calcium and phosphorus. The whole plant is used.

Uses - Treatment for all gastric weaknesses and ailments, nerves and neuralgia, female ailments including failing milk supply, allergies, bronchitis, anemia, bruises, colitis, coughs, diabetes, fever, flu, hay fever, headache, migraines, lung problems, sinus congestion, ulcers, reduces inflammation, has a reputation for stimulating and developing breasts.

Externally - It can be used as a poultice for relief of abscess, boils, tumors and running sores.

Caution - Avoid during pregnancy as it can be a uterine stimulant.

Feverfew

Actions - Anti-inflammatory, vasodilator, relaxant, digestive bitter, uterine stimulant.

It is one of the most important aids for female ailments the plant exerting remarkable powers over the uterus, the whole plant is used. Has a good reputation for migraine headaches, may help with arthritis when it is in the inflammatory stage, painful periods. Feverfew inhibits the manufacture of substances causing inflammation.

Uses - Digestive aid and tonic, treatment for all female irregularities especially scanty or failing menses, inflamed or weak uterus and uterine and vaginal ulcers, abortion, difficult labor, retained afterbirth, arthritis, inflammations.

Cautions - Do not use during pregnancy because of the stimulant action on the womb. The fresh leaves may cause mouth ulcers in sensitive people.

Figwort

Actions - Alterative, diuretic, mild purgative, heart stimulant.

Used for any skin condition where there is itching and irritation. This herb cleans out the system especially the blood and bowels. Can be used has a heart stimulant or for poor circulation but is contraindicated for this when there is a rapid heartbeat (tachycardia)

Uses - Failing or weak heart, eczema, psoriasis, acne, cradle cap, mild laxative. Externally use for boils, burns ,eczema, rashes, ringworm and wounds.

Fumitory

Actions - Diuretic, cholagogue, laxative, alterative.

Has a long history of use in the treatment of skin problems such as eczema and acne, its action is probably due to a general cleansing mediated via the kidneys and liver. Cows and sheep seek it out greedily. The whole plant is used.

Uses - All forms of liver ailments and gallbladder problems, skin eruptions, eczema, wounds, scabies, ulcerated mouth, inflamed liver, jaundice, biliousness.

Garlic

Actions - Immune stimulant, anti-bacterial, anti-viral, anti-fungal, anti-septic, anti-oxidant, diaphoretic, cholagogue, hypotensive, anti-spasmodic, vermifuge and many more.

The plant is rich in volatile oil and sulphur and because of its remarkable penetrating, disinfecting and mucous expelling powers garlic is a valuable basic remedy for the treatment of all ailments in which the cleansing of the blood stream and expulsion of mucous accumulations is required. Garlic can be used to prevent and treat respiratory infections. Anyone who has had garlic breath has experienced this herb's aromatic compounds being excreted through their lungs which is why garlic's active ingredients can be so effective for respiratory complaints. Garlic is extremely effective in dissolving and cleansing cholesterol from the blood stream, it stimulates the digestive tract, kills worms, parasites and harmful bacteria, normalizes blood pressure, reduces fever, gas and cramps.

Uses- All infections, coughs, colds, flu, bronchitis, all fevers, pulmonary conditions, gastric and skin complaints, rheumatism, all worms and also liver fluke, mange, ringworm, ticks and lice.

Acts on Bacteria, Viruses and Internal Parasites.

Externally - You can use garlic for ring worm and ear ache, to disinfect wounds and sores, parasitical infections.

Guaiacum

Actions - Anti rheumatic, anti-inflammatory, laxative, diaphoretic, diuretic, alterative, peripheral circulatory stimulant.

Specific for rheumatic complaints with lots of inflammation, aids in the treatment of gout and can be used here as a preventative. Care must be taken with this herb especially in allergic conditions.

Gentian

Actions - Bitter, gastric stimulant, sialagogue, cholagogue.

The root is the medicinal part. Gentian is one of the most important tonic herbs being considered the Prince of the Bitters. Quells vomiting when all other herbs fail, promotes the production of saliva, gastric juices and bile along with stimulating peristalsis, indicated where there is a lack of appetite and sluggishness of the digestive system.

Uses - Treatment of all forms of digestive weakness, vomiting, nervous ailments including hysteria, malaria, to improve the appetite of all poor feeders.

Ginger

Actions- Carminative, anti-inflammatory, vasodilator, circulatory stimulant, diaphoretic, anti-emetic.

The therapeutic benefits of ginger are largely due to its volatile oil and oleoresin content. Ginger is an excellent remedy for many digestive complaints, including nausea, colic, wind and indigestion. Its antiseptic properties also make it beneficial for gastro-intestinal infections. For the older, arthritic horse, ginger is a useful maintenance herb. It stimulates the circulatory system and helps blood flow and increases stamina. Aids in fighting colds, colitis, digestive disorders, wind, increases saliva.

Uses- Indigestion, nausea, feverish conditions especially when chills are present, travel sickness especially sea sickness, dyspepsia, colic, flatulence.

Caution - Don't use large doses on a empty stomach.

Ginkgo Biloba

Actions - Anti fungal, anti-bacterial, antioxidant, anti-tussive, astringent, expectorant, anti-allergy and anti-inflammatory but mainly used for its Peripheral Vaso - Dilator effects.

Is native to Northern China and is considered the world's oldest tree species. This herb can be helpful for a horse resuming work after a spell, or for older horses that are sound for riding but are slowing down. Due to its effect on peripheral and cerebral (brain) circulation it can assist the blood supply to limbs, and general alertness. (think of mixing with Hawthorn). The leading symptoms pointing to Ginkgo are cold hands and feet. This herb opens up the femoral arteries and neck arteries increasing blood supply to those areas thus improving the function of everything in those areas by the increase in oxygen and blood sugar. For the old animal thinking and seeing may improve and walking may also become a bit easier. In asthma ginkgo helps reduce the inflammation response making the attacks less severe. The herb is safe to use as a tonic. This is a good herb to take in a mixed antioxidant formula.

Ginseng (Panax)

Actions - Anti depressive, restorative, tonic, adaptogen, stimulating adrenal agent, increases resistance and improves mental and physical performance.

This is the strong ginseng, think twice about giving it to a horse with a shy and sensitive nature its more for the outgoing and competitive nature. This herb can help with depression especially when caused by debility and exhaustion. It can be used in general for exhaustion and weakness. Used to increase mental and physical performance, to improve concentration, vigilance and work efficiency, stamina, for combating internal or external stress factors of any kind - athletics, endurance activities, aging, surgery, disease, infections, cold, but especially degenerative conditions and problems of old age. This is a good herb for infertility.

Cautions - Avoid with high blood pressure, during acute infections. This herb can be over stimulating for some. Use month on month off.

Ginseng Siberian

Actions - Adaptogen, vaso dilator, increases stamina, circulatory stimulant.

This herb is very similar to the one above but is a milder version and can be used all the time as it does not build up in the system like Panax Ginseng. Always consider giving a break from herbs as it is not good to use any herb all the time except maybe Hawthorn for a failing heart.

Goldenrod

Actions - Ant catarrhal, anti-inflammatory, antiseptic, diaphoretic, carminative, diuretic, astringent, tonic, hypotensive.

It is famed as a wound herb, is a important remedy for female disorders, all cattle eat it and it brings them into good appetite and gives bloom, the whole plant is used, traditionally used for inflammation, upper respiratory catarrh, use with other herbs for influenza, flatulent dyspepsia, as a urinary anti-inflammatory and anti-septic, cystitis, urethritis and also used for urinary stones. This herb is also used for arthritis.

Uses - A powerful digestive aid, treatment of jaundice, kidney problems.

Externally - For wounds, to stop bleeding, cleansing gangrenous conditions.

Gravel Root

Actions - Diuretic, anti-lithic, anti-rheumatic.

Used primarily for kidney stones and gravel. In urinary infections such as cystitis and urethritis it may be used with benefit, good in the systemic treatment of rheumatism and gout.

Grindelia

Actions - Antispasmodic, expectorant, hypotensive, cardiac relaxant, diuretic, tonic.

This plant comes from the Americas and has long been used for asthma, it acts to relax the smooth muscles and is good for asthma and bronchitis especially when these are associated with a rapid heartbeat and a nervous disposition. Also used for whooping cough and respiratory catarrh. Ellingwood a famous Herbalist from the past considered it a specific for asthmatic breathing. Because of the relaxing effect on the heart and pulse there may be a lowering of blood pressure. Has a tonic effect on the lungs and kidneys and is mildly diuretic.

Topically this herb has been used for eczema, insect bites, poison ivy and burns.

Caution - Don't use for those with weak hearts or low blood pressure.

Hawthorn

Actions - Cardiac tonic, hypotensive, adaptogen.

Strengthens the muscles and nerves of the heart, aids in relieving emotional stress, regulates high and low blood pressure, helps combat arteriosclerosis and heart disease. With regard to horses, hawthorn's affects on peripheral circulation makes it valuable for treating conditions such as navicular and laminitis. Indeed, horses and ponies suffering from these ailments have been observed seeking out the new growth on hawthorn bushes. This is more of a balancing herb, if the blood pressure is high or low the herb will balance it if the electrical activity is playing up with rapid or erratic heart beat it will try to balance it. Strengthens and helps to remove plaques from the blood vessels. This is a herb for taking in the long term.

Uses - As a tonic to the circulatory system and to strengthen the heart.

Hops

Actions - Sedative, hypnotic, antiseptic, astringent, nervine, bitter digestive tonic, antibacterial.

Famed for its tonic and nervine properties, pain reliever, sleep inducer, anti-septic, vermifuge, tension that leads to restlessness, headache, indigestion, and mucous colitis. Good for when digestive problems are caused by worry or nerves. Good for nervous horses. One of the main remedies for IBS. Acts on the central nervous system and calms and eases anxiety. Hops contains estrogenic substances which could interfere with hormone therapy.

Uses - Treatment of all digestive ailments, general debility, failing appetite, wasting, fevers, eczema, worms, to quietens restless animals.

Externally - Eczema.

Horehound (White)

Actions - Expectorant, anti-spasmodic, bitter, digestive, vulnerary.

Is one of the most important pectoral herbs a famed cough and throat remedy, the bitter action stimulates the flow of bile and thus improves digestion.

Uses - Treatment of cough, pneumonia, pleurisy, bronchitis, TB, atrophy of the lungs, ear disorders, canker, diarrhea, inflammation of the liver, jaundice.

Horse Chestnut

Actions - Circulatory tonic, astringent, anti-inflammatory, nutritive.

Has a action on the vessels of the circulatory system especially veins where it seems to increase their strength and tone. Can be used internally and externally on the veins themselves. The nuts in the past were fed to animals as a tonic food and was also said to enrich the milk. It also was used in the past to treat the cough of horses and this is where it gets its name.

Uses - Inflammation of veins, varicose veins, piles, capillary weakness

Cautions - Avoid with kidney disease.

Horseradish

Actions - Stimulant, carminative, mild laxative, diuretic, antiseptic, tonic.

It's hot properties make it valuable in expelling worms, stimulating appetite and as a general tonic, it is a internal antiseptic, helps to remove excess urine from the system and stones from the bladder, urinary infection, all parts of the plant are used, can be used in influenza and fevers, eases wind and gripping pains in the digestive system, bronchitis.

Uses - Worm and kidney treatment, to reduce tumors, asthma, bronchitis, sinusitis, remedy for lack of appetite and over thinness.

Externally - As a poultice for swellings.

Horsetail

Actions - Astringent, diuretic, vulnerary.

Goats eat the plant but it is not a good food for cows, excellent astringent for the genito-urinary system reducing bleeding and healing wounds thanks to its high silica content, inflammation of the prostrate, tones and astringes the urinary system making it a good remedy for incontinence and bed wetting. Use for kidney stones as the high silica content erodes stones. May speed up the healing of bone, flesh and cartilage due to its high mineral content.

Uses - Nasal hemorrhage, laryngitis, intestinal ulcer, inflammation of the uterus, vagina and bladder, dysentery, enlarged anal glands, obesity, dropsy, a strong dose dissolves stones in the bladder.

Caution - If used over a long period it may decrease vitamin B1.

Hypericum (St John's Wort)

Actions - Anti-inflammatory, astringent, anti-viral, anti-spasmodic, nervine, vulnerary, antibacterial.

The name St John's Wort came from the Knights of St John of Jerusalem who used the herb to treat battle wounds.

Uses - Taken internally has a sedative and pain reducing effect, neuralgic pain, anxiety, tension, rheumatic pain, sciatica, for pains that shoot along the nerves, as a lotion it will speed the healing of wounds and bruises and is used where there is damage to the nerve rich areas, varicose veins and mild burns. Good for inflamed joints and rheumatic pain. In humans recently the herb has become popular to use as a antidepressant especially for cases of anxiety. Use as a lotion on wounds especially in the nerve rich areas such as the lips and fingers. As a lotion it is commonly mixed with Calendula, Homoeopaths call this lotion Hypercal.

Caution - Animals that overdose on Hypericum become photosensitive and have to be locked in the barn for a while so as not to become sun burnt.

Hyssop

Actions - Anti spasmodic, expectorant, antiviral, nervine, diaphoretic, sedative, carminative.

A important plant in pectoral complaints because it removes mucous accumulations and also tones up the membranes and fortifies the whole system along with being a respiratory antiviral. Is a mild vermifuge the Nordic countries use it as a vermifuge for delicate lambs and kids. Coughs, bronchitis, chronic catarrh, colds and flu's, anxiety states, hysteria, petit mal.

Uses - Treatment of cough especially the more spasmodic coughs such as whooping, sore throat, pneumonia, pleurisy, TB, or any respiratory disease, worms, eye disorders, conjunctivitis.

Juniper

Actions - Diuretic, antiseptic, carminative, anti-rheumatic.

The whole plant is a tonic and nerve stimulant, excellent antiseptic in conditions like cystitis, stimulating to the kidney nephrons (avoid in kidney disease), the bitter action aids digestion and eases flatulent colic.

Uses - Treatment of inflamed liver and kidneys, gallstones, jaundice, obesity, sciatica, rheumatism, blood ailments, acid milk, malaria.

Caution - Avoid in kidney disease. Avoid in pregnancy.

Kelp

Actions - Antihypothyroid, anti-rheumatic, nutritive,

Used mainly for under active thyroid (iodine) especially when it is thought to be the cause of overweight. Helps in the relief of rheumatism internally and externally. Added to feed for nutrition. Can be used to slim fat horses. Make sure that iodine isn't in any of the supplements you are already giving. It is good for coat and hoof conditions.

Ladys Mantle

Actions - Astringent, diuretic, anti-inflammatory, emmenagogue, vulnerary.

This herb has a affinity to the womb where it helps with pain, bleeding and getting the cycle back to normal. Horses, goats and sheep seek out the herb, the plant is tonic and an important fortifier for the blood and walls of the arteries, it is a old herbal remedy for diabetes, reduces period pains and excessive bleeding, diarrhea, sores, ulcers a good menopause herb.

Uses - Treatment for lack of appetite, wasting, weak blood, sluggish blood, all weaknesses of the arteries, heart disease, taken from one period to another it is reputed to aid conception in barren animals.

Lemon Balm (Melissa)

Actions - Carminative, antispasmodic, anti-depressive, diaphoretic, hypotensive, emmenagogue, nervine, rejuvenating tonic, Anti-viral.

In the past this plant was used to attract bees by rubbing it all around a new hive and the smell made the bees want to stay. The name Melissa is Greek for honey bee. The Arabs say it gives intelligence to any animal that feeds upon it.

Relieves spasms in the digestive tract and is used in flatulent dyspepsia. Good for digestive problems brought on from worry, anxiety and stress. Has a tonic effect on the heart and circulatory system causing mild vasodilatation of the peripheral blood vessels which can help to lower blood pressure and also may calm the electrical activity of the heart. Has also been used in animals for retained afterbirth and as a anti-viral for infections such as herpes.

Caution - Can sometimes lower thyroid function.

Licorice

Actions - Expectorant, demulcent, anti-inflammatory, adrenal agent, anti-spasmodic, mild laxative.

The root part is used , possessing unique pectoral and emollient properties, it is also nutritive and slightly laxative, It contains the building blocks of hormones, has a marked effect on the endocrine system, catarrh, gastric and peptic ulcers, abdominal colic. Its ability to soothe irritated mucous membranes and to break up phlegm and ease coughing sees licorice employed in respiratory conditions, coughing, bronchitis, and chest colds. Can be used for treating inflammatory and allergic conditions.. Licorice has effects on the adrenal glands which are protective, restorative, tonic and stimulatory. These properties can aid the horse which is recovering from steroid therapy or abuse.

Uses - Treatment of cough, inflamed throat, pneumonia, pleurisy, TB, all catarrhal conditions, gallstones, chronic constipation, mild worms in young animals, female infertility, pains of colic.

Caution - Do not use with high blood pressure. Long term use depletes potassium which raises the blood pressure. Don't use with steroids.

Lime Blossom (Linden)

Actions - Nervine, antispasmodic, diaphoretic, diuretic, mild astringent.

Possesses powerful nervine and blood cleansing properties, used for fits and nervous twitching of all kinds including epilepsy, a good tonic for bees, nervous tension, as a prophylactic against arteriosclerosis, migraines, feverish colds and flu.

Uses - Treatment of all nervous ailments especially epilepsy, twitching, vertigo, good for colds and to remove the slime and mucous from the system, treatment of vomiting, heart pains, fevers, treatment of tumors by poultice.

Marsh Mallow

Actions - Demulcent, anti-inflammatory, expectorant, astringent.

Its therapeutic effects are largely due to its significant mucilage and pectin content, aided by its anti-inflammatory properties. The foliage of the mallow is eaten by all animals, the roots are the main part used for internal medicine and also the leaves which are especially used for inflammation of the stomach and bowel and especially used for ulcers, it contains over half its weight in sweet tasting mucilage which possess unique properties of lubricating, soothing and healing. A poultice can be used for all inflammatory conditions. Horses who have colic, or who are scouring, can benefit from the soothing and healing effects of marshmallow also see Slippery Elm. Consider using as a supplement for horses prone to colic and ulcers. Marshmallow can also be used to soothe inflamed and irritated mucous membranes of the respiratory and urinary systems. Dry coughs, sore throats, urinary tract inflammation and cystitis have all been relieved by the effects of marshmallow.

Uses - Treatment of sore throats, pulmonary catarrhs, pleurisy, cystitis, diarrhea, dysentery, ulcers, bowel inflammations and hemorrhages.

Externally - All skin eruptions, abrasions, swellings, inflammations, bruises, sore inflamed udders.

Marigold see Calendula

Meadowsweet

Actions - Anti-inflammatory, anti-rheumatic, antacid, anti-emetic, stomachic, astringent.

A important fever and diarrhea herb, the gypsies use as a spring tonic for their animals, eaten plentifully by goats and sheep, acts to protect and soothe the mucous membranes of the digestive tract reducing excess acidity and easing nausea, heart burn, hyperacidity, gastritis, peptic ulcers. This herb is a good acid balancer and is good for correcting over acid systems. Meadowsweet is the forerunner of aspirin as this is the first herb it was synthesized from in 1835 but as this herb contains its own buffering agents it is gentle on the stomach. Used to help reduce inflammation and for pain relief in case of arthritic conditions. Useful alone or in combination with other herbs for effective pain management.

Uses - Fevers, arthritis, diarrhea and the above mentioned.

Caution - Avoid if sensitive to salicylates.

Mistletoe

Actions - Nervine, hypotensive, cardiac depressant, possibly anti tumor.

It will quiet soothe and tone the nervous system, acts directly on the vagus nerve to reduce heart rate while strengthening the walls of the peripheral capillaries, reduces blood pressure and eases arteriosclerosis, nervous tachycardia, headache due to high blood pressure.

Uses - Treatment of nervous ailments, epilepsy, hysteria, heart tonic, uterine and vaginal bleeding.

Milk Thistle - St Mary's Thistle

Actions - Cholagogue, galactagogue, demulcent.

This herb is said to rejuvenate the liver, for problems like hepatitis it is used alone at first as it drains the liver probably by its action of stimulating the gallbladder to release bile. Much of the therapeutic benefit of the seeds is attributed to a group of potent antioxidant bioflavonoids, known together as silymarin, which are able to guard and stabilize cell membranes, preventing the invasion of toxins, as well as enhance the regeneration of liver cells already damaged by detoxification processes. for horses who have suffered liver damage from poisons, infections, high worm burdens, reactions to worming drugs, or excessive drug use. Can be taken long term and needs be taken for a prolonged period at least 4-12 weeks to be of most benefit In disease like hepatitis you just use it by itself sometimes for months after this time you can consider adding Dandelion.

Used to increase milk production in mothers and for gallbladder problems.

Uses - Liver problems, gallbladder problems, hepatitis, to increase milk production.

Milk Thistle and Dandelion Together

Actions of Milk Thistle - Cholagogue, galactagogue, demulcent.

Known as the liver regenerator.

Milk Thistle and dandelion together make a good and gentle liver cleanser, detoxifier and repairer. Use for liver or kidney damage, hepatitis (include Echinacea), jaundice, leptospirosis and parvo virus recovery. It may be helpful in chronic skin disorders, tumors and cancer. This is a major antioxidant. Pets that have been on a lot of veterinary drugs, heart worm prevention, vaccinations, de-worming drugs or chemotherapy need this healing from these herbs.

Motherwort

Actions - Sedative, emmenagogue, antispasmodic, cardiac tonic.
As its species name indicates, it has long been considered a nerve and heart remedy. It strengthens heart function, particularly where it is weak. Antispasmodic and sedative, the herb causes relaxation rather than drowsiness. Motherwort is considered a life giving plant, beneficial for all female disorders and a general heart tonic. Delayed or suppressed menses especially where anxiety or tension are involved, specific for over rapid heartbeat brought on by anxiety or tension, lowers high blood pressure and is used for the pains of birth and given for a few days after so as to prevent bleeding and infection.

Mullein

Actions - Expectorant, demulcent, mild diuretic, mild sedative, vulnerary.
The herb is famed for its powers in pulmonary ailments being much used in lung ailments of cattle, a bone flesh and cartilage builder, aids in healing respiratory ailments, asthma, bronchitis, sinus congestion, soothing to any inflammation and relieves pain, acts to relieve spasms and clears the lungs, tones mucous membranes of the respiratory system, inflammation of the trachea, painful coughs. The leaves of Mullein were traditionally fed to animals that cough especially horses.
Uses - Coughs, pneumonia, bronchitis, pleurisy, TB, asthma, diarrhea, internal bleeding of the lung and bowel.

Myrrh

Actions - Anti microbial, astringent, carminative, anti-catarrhal, expectorant, vulnerary, Antiseptic, antifungal, alterative.

Stimulates production of white blood cells and also has a good anti-microbial action so this is a good herb for immune boosting and fighting diseases.

Uses - Stomach viruses, coughs, asthma, infections of the mouth, mouth ulcers, gingivitis, sinusitis, laryngitis.

Externally - Healing and antiseptic to wounds and abrasions.

Cautions - Use only in small amounts for short periods. Large amounts can speed heartbeat.

Nasturtium

Actions - Anti microbial, expectorant, anthelmintic.

The plant has a hot biting character especially in the seeds which were once used to make a popular pickle. Animals eat the whole plant greedily. The seeds of this plant are collected and used on poultry as a wormer. The seeds can be preserved in vinegar and used as a tonic and anti-worm remedy. A powerful anti-microbial especially when used locally on bacterial infections. Internally use for infections more so in the respiratory system such as bronchitis, flu and colds where it is used in breaking up congestion in the respiratory passages.

Uses - Bacterial infections, respiratory infections, as a tonic, poor sight, worms. Locally as a general antiseptic.

Neem

Actions - Anti-inflammatory, alterative, antibacterial, antiviral, antifungal, anthelmintic, bitter tonic, immune stimulant.

The name in Sanskrit means curer of all ailments and another name it is called is village pharmacy. Its antibacterial properties are good for Staph and Clostridia, Neem effectively kills lice and is good for topical applications to skin problems.

Uses - Ring worm, eczema, rash, arthritis and rheumatism and is used for malaria. Use as a wash for ticks, mites, scabies and fleas.

Cautions - Not for use for infants and the elderly and not for long term internal use.

Nettles

Actions - Astringent, diuretic, galactagogue, tonic, nutritive.

Nettle is perhaps best known as a highly nutritious feed herb/fodder for animals, and has been used through the ages for this purpose. It is considered a spring tonic and detoxifier for human and animal alike. One of the richest sources of chlorophyll in the vegetable kingdom, rich in iron, lime, sodium, Vit C, chlorine and contains much protein. Preventative against many ailments, increases milk yield, fattener for poultry. Good astringent for stopping bleeding anywhere but especially in the urinary tract. Good for eczema in the young especially in the nervous young. Good for pregnant and nursing mothers. The seeds can be used as a thyroid tonic.

Uses - Treatment of wasting diseases, poor appetite, lung disorders, blood impurities, worms, fever, cold, hay fever, allergies, eczema, diarrhea, hemorrhage.

Externally - Paralysis, rheumatism, arthritis, loss of muscular power.

Caution - Only buy the product prepared for herbal use.

Oats

Actions - Nerve tonic, anti-depressant, nutritive, demulcent, vulnerary.

Oats are a strength giving cereal low in starch high in mineral content especially potassium, phosphorus, magnesium and calcium and also the B vitamins. Is a nerve tonic and bone builder used for nervous debility, nervous exhaustion, general debility, skin conditions.

Uses - As a nutritive food, remedy and cure for rickets, important for strong teeth, hooves, horns, nails and hair.

Parsley

Actions - Diuretic, carminative, emmenagogue, expectorant.

Well-liked by sheep and goats, improves their milk yield and keeps them free from foot ills. It is a great enricher of the blood being very rich in iron and copper. Nutrient, digestive tract tonic, diuretic, high in potassium minerals and vitamins, bladder and kidney infections, incontinence, blood cleanser, immune builder, tonic for the blood vessels, aids in afterbirth pains, mainly used as a diuretic, carminative and emmenagogue. Is a good source of chlorophyll, parsley is useful for combating bad breath. Its diuretic properties are beneficial in: arthritic/rheumatic conditions associated with poor kidney function; urinary infections; kidney and bladder stones. Parsley also acts as a digestive tonic by easing spasms and minimizing flatulence.

Uses - Treatment of all disorders of the kidneys and bladder, gravel, stones, congestion, cystitis, jaundice, obesity, dropsy, worms, rheumatism, prostrate problems, sciatica, swellings of the joints, the root can be used for constipation and obstructions of the intestines.

Caution - Do not use in pregnancy.

Passion Flower Incarnata

Actions - Sedative, antispasmodic, anodyne, relaxant, epilepsy, shingles, asthma, hypotensive.

A good herb for insomnia and a very effective herb for nerve pains especially in conditions like shingles. This herbs focus is more on restlessness and irritability, hysteria and anxiety and is soothing to the mentally worried and overworked it acts on nervousness especially due to unrest, agitation, worry, exhaustion and cerebral excitement. Can be of benefit to horses that are generally nervous and apprehensive. Used in the treatment of convulsions, epilepsy, tremors, hypertension, nervous breakdowns, migraines and neuralgias.

Cautions - Large doses may cause nausea and vomiting. Do not use while pregnant.

Pau D'Arco

Actions - Alterative, anodyne, analgesic, antifungal, antibacterial, anti-inflammatory, antioxidant, antiviral, diuretic, immune stimulant. This herb comes from Brazil and is used by the Indians there. It possesses properties that are antibiotic, tumor inhibiting, virus killing, anti-fungal and anti-malarial. Builds up the immune system. It's anti-inflammatory action applies especially in the stomach and intestines as well as for conditions such as cystitis, inflammation of the cervix, arthritis and prostatitis, it is a good herb for fighting fungal infections while building up the immune system. This herb is used for lung, colon and prostate cancer. It contains a chemical called lapachol that inhibits tumor cell growth by preventing them from metabolizing oxygen. Pau D'Arco also lowers blood sugar levels and acts as a mild laxative.

Pennyroyal

Actions - Carminative, diaphoretic, stimulant, emmenagogue, insecticide.

The forerunner of the cultivated mints, animals seek it for its tonic and stimulating properties, herdsmen use it after calving as a stimulant and restorative to the cow, abdominal colic due to wind, spasmodic pain, eases anxiety, its main use is as a emmenagogue to stimulate the menstrual process and strengthen uterine contractions. Helpful against nausea and nervous conditions.

Uses - Treatment of digestive ailments including failing appetite, sour stomach and internal gas, cough, pneumonia, fever, bronchitis and pleurisy, after birth exhaustion, female complaints.

Externally used as a insect repellant (oil) and a lotion for itching skin eg rashes, psoriasis etc.

Caution - Do not use in pregnancy or in large doses.

Peppermint

Actions - Carminative, diaphoretic, anti-spasmodic, anti-emetic, nervine, analgesic, anti-septic.

Best known for its ability to aid digestion and relieve gastrointestinal distress. Peppermint owes most of its medicinal value to menthol, which is cooling, anesthetic, antiseptic and soothing to the stomach. For horses, peppermint's aroma is useful for tempting fussy eaters and/or helping to mask the smell of less pleasant herbs in their feed. It eases flatulence/bloating, increases the flow of bile from the liver and relaxes both gastrointestinal spasms and tight skeletal muscles.

Uses- Nausea, heartburn, indigestion, colic, flatulence, dyspepsia, vomiting, fevers, migraine headaches and irritable bowel syndrome (IBS) and for travel sickness think of adding Ginger for this.

Caution - May reduce milk flow if breast feeding.

Plantain

Actions - Expectorant, demulcent, astringent, antibacterial, diuretic. Goats and sheep enjoy its foliage and poultry seek out the seeds. Plantain clears heat and removes excess fluid from the body while at the same time soothing inflammation and irritated tissues. The whole plant yields soothing mucilage similar to linseed, gentle expectorant while soothing sore and inflamed membranes, coughs, bronchitis etc. Its astringency aids in diarrhea and cystitis where there is bleeding. Is good for using in the treatment of stomach ulcers and has been used for blood poisoning. The plant is high in chlorophyll and good for use on wounds.

Uses - Treatment of dysentery, hemorrhages, internal obstructions and ulcers, fevers.

Externally - Wounds, sores, ulcers and all bites, eye disorders.

Poke Root - Phytolacca

Actions - Purgative, emetic, stimulant, anti-rheumatic and anti-catarrhal.

May be seen primarily as a remedy for use in infections of the upper respiratory tract removing catarrh and aiding in the cleansing of the lymphatic glands, it may be used for catarrh, tonsillitis, laryngitis and swollen glands. It will be found to be of value to problems elsewhere in the body involving the lymphatic system especially mastitis (Homoeopathic form works faster). Also used in long standing cases of rheumatism. Poke Root stimulates the immune system by increasing T cell activity. Care must be taken with this herb as in large doses it is a powerful emetic and purgative. Can be used as a lotion in mastitis. This herb in the past has been known as cancer root and has been used for breast cancer and tumors.

Uses - Mastitis and other lymphatic problems.

External Use - Breast cancer, tumors, mastitis, boils, fungal infections, shingles, psoriasis, scabies and eczema.

Cautions - This is a very strong herb so use it very carefully in small doses.

Raspberry

Actions - Astringent, tonic, refrigerant, parturient.

Raspberry leaf has been used for mares with oestrus problems and the attendant behavioral disturbances. For mares that have had or may have difficulty conceiving it can be given for a period prior to mating. Generally, raspberry leaf is used to tone the uterine muscles, encourage an easy labor, and hemorrhaging during and after birth Highly tonic and cleansing improving the condition of the organism during pregnancy ensuring speedy and strong expulsion of the fetus at birth, use as a drench in retained afterbirth, acclaimed as a tonic for male animals and as a cure for sterility, becomes especially potent for female use when blended with feverfew - 3 parts to 1 part of feverfew. As a astringent it can be used in diarrhea and leucorrhoea, it is valuable in easing mouth problems such as mouth ulcers, bleeding gums and inflammations

Uses - Prevention and treatment of all female ailments, retained afterbirth, digestive ailments including diarrhea, treatment of mouth and throat ailments as a gargle.

Red Clover

Actions - Alterative, diuretic, expectorant, antispasmodic, nutritive.

The flowers are a powerful tonic and a cure for nervous twitches, wasting bodies and cough. The whole plant is sedative. Good for treating conditions like eczema and psoriasis and other chronic skin conditions. In the respiratory system we can use the actions of expectorant and antispasmodic to treat conditions such as bronchitis, whooping cough and maybe the eczema and asthma syndrome and as this herb seems to have a affinity for the throat we could use it for tonsillitis to. In the nervous system we can use the antispasmodic action to treat stress and nervousness along with hypertension. The alterative action of this herb helps to clean out the body and makes this herbs action on the skin very effective and it is probably this action that makes it useful in cancers especially breast and Ovary cancer. The herb has proved beneficial in cancers of the stomach and throat. This herb is in a lot of female formulas now because they extract the Isoflavones (Plant Hormones) from it and it is said to be very rich in these.

Uses - Tonic, treatment for general debility, weak nerves, throat ailments, cancers, tumors, detox, skin diseases and respiratory problems.

Rose Hips

Actions - Nutrient, mild laxative, mild diuretic, mild astringent.
The foliage is enjoyed by all animals. The flowers are tonic and astringent. The fruits are slightly aperient and rich in vitamin C. A good spring tonic and aid to general debility and exhaustion. Used to fight infection and curb stress. Rosehips are often fed to horses recuperating from injury as they help to restore the immune system and aid tissue repair and leaking capillaries with their bioflavonoids.

Rosemary

Actions - Carminative, aromatic, antispasmodic, anti-depressive, antiseptic, parasiticide.
It imparts a fine fragrance and tonic properties to the milk of goat and sheep which graze it eagerly. The powdered form is used on wounds as a antiseptic, nerve tonic, carminative, insecticide, acts as a circulatory and nerve stimulant, headache.

Uses - Treatment of all ailments of the heart, rheumatism, fits, epilepsy, paralysis, gastritis, diarrhea, dysentery.

Externally - Wounds, falling hair and nervous spasms.

Caution - Excessive large doses can poison and cause death.

Rue

Actions - Antispasmodic, emmenagogue, anti tussive, abortifacient.

The essential principal of the plant is Rutin which possesses most potent powers strengthening weakened blood vessels, toning the nerves and glands and imparting hardness to bones teeth and nails, highly antiseptic and is also a insecticide, it is also an old remedy for the prevention and cure of rabies. Regulates menses, used to bring on suppressed menses, the anti-spasmodic action is used to relax smooth muscles especially in the digestive system where it will ease gripping and bowel tension, spasmodic coughs, lowers elevated blood pressure.

Uses - Treatment of fevers, epilepsy, neuralgia, heart disease, ailments of the arteries and veins, worms, all skin parasites including scabies and ringworm,.

Caution - Avoid in pregnancy.

Reshi Mushroom

Actions - Immune stimulant, antibacterial, anti-tumor, adaptogen, rejuvenative, anti-inflammatory

As a immune stimulant it helps to activate the phagocytosis of macrophages and may increase interferon. Aids in the prevention of illness as well as in recovery. Helps normalize blood pressure reduces cholesterol and can inhibit histamine release. Inhibits the inflammation associated with allergies, bronchitis, conjunctivitis and rheumatism. Good for treating chronic hepatitis. Good for over overcoming fatigue, anxiety and stress while improving stamina at the same time.

Uses - Good as a all-round immune booster and restorative tonic. Works well with its fellow mushroom Shitake as they tend to complement each others actions and together they can be used to attack acute viral diseases. In chronic disease use 1/10 of the recommended dose.

Shitake Mushroom

Actions - Immune stimulant, antiviral, rejuvinative, aphrodisiac.

Animal studies have shown a antiviral and anti-tumor activity as well as the stimulation of killer T cells. Shitake enhances the stem cells in the bone marrow to create more B and T cells. Lowers blood pressure by helping the body get rid of excessive salt and can be used in AIDs like diseases. Stimulates the production of interferon and provides significant protection against type A Viruses which causes epidemic influenza.

Uses - Good as a all-round immune booster and restorative tonic. Works well with its fellow mushroom Reshi as they tend to complement each other's actions and together they can be used to attack acute viral diseases. In chronic disease use 1/10 of the recommended dose.

Sage

Actions - Carminative, antispasmodic, antiseptic, astringent.

Sage is well liked by animals and as with other aromatics makes the milk refreshing, tonic and increases the milk yield, it is a nervine, digestive and blood cleanser, a first rate remedy for all disorders of the throat, lungs and ears, inflamed and bleeding gums, inflamed tongue or general mouth inflammation, mouth ulcers, a good mouth wash.

Uses - Treatment of nerve debility, paralysis, all gastric ailments, constipation, obesity and female ailments, eczema, fevers, wound infections.

Dose - For horses infuse 1 teaspoon of powdered herb in 2 cups of water. Use in small doses. For sore mouths and throat ailments give mixed with honey.

Caution - Stimulates the muscles of the uterus so should be avoided during pregnancy.

Sarsaparilla

Actions - Alterative, diuretic, diaphoretic, anti-rheumatic, tonic.

Has a purifying effect on the genito urinary tract helping in the clearing of infections and the excretion of uric acid. Has chemicals and properties that aid in the production of testosterone, eliminates poisons and toxins from the blood and helps clean the system, useful in scaling skin conditions such as psoriasis, used in rheumatism and arthritis.

Uses - Rheumatism, arthritis, gout, skin eruptions, ringworm, internal inflammations, colds, catarrh.

Slippery Elm Bark Powder

Actions - Demulcent, emollient, nutrient, astringent.

Slippery elm bark provides a nutritious gruel which also possesses remarkable medicinal properties acting as a poultice both internally and externally. A nutrient and food for very old or young or weak especially if mixed with honey, coats and heals all inflamed tissues internally and externally and is used for the stomach, intestines, ulcers, ulcerative colitis, enteritis, dysentery, constipation and internal bleeding of the digestive tract.

Uses - Treatment of all digestive complaints especially ulcers for which it is a specific, dysentery, all pectoral disorders including TB, lung and bronchial hemorrhage, wasting diseases, rickets, stunted growth. Calves with scour can be kept alive on this mixed with honey while the non treated can die.

Externally - A poultice for all skin ailments especially old ailments and hard swellings.

Shepherds Purse

Actions - Uterine stimulant, astringent, diuretic.

Possesses important astringent properties, all animals like this herb and poultry seek it eagerly.

A gentle diuretic, diarrhea, wounds, reduces excessive menstruation.

Uses - Treatment of hemorrhages internal and external, profuse bleeding of deep wounds, kidney ailments, female problems.

Skullcap

Actions - Nervine tonic, sedative, antispasmodic.

Supreme nerve herb and has restored many cases of nervous disorders, nervous tension, seizures, epilepsy, PMS, carminative nervine and nervous system repairer, pain reliever, spinal problems, twitching muscles, rheumatism, high blood pressure, restlessness, nervous heart conditions.

Uses - Treatment of all nervous complaints especially hysteria, fits, meningitis, nervous spasms, gastroenteritis, an old cure for rabies.

St John's Wort see Hypericum

Sweet Violets

Actions - Alterative, expectorant, anti-inflammatory, anti-cancer, diuretic, antifungal, antiseptic.

Is used with Red Clover as a detoxifier and a blood cleanser. Especially useful to animals that have had a toxic reaction to Vaccination. Good for coughs and bronchitis. Can be used as a poultice on cancer tumors.

Uses - Skin problems, tumors, warts, behavior reactions or other aggravations from vaccination, digestive disorders, seizures, cancer, cysts, boils, abscesses, chronic skin diseases.

Senna Pods

Actions - Cathartic

One of the most important laxatives because it is also a cleanser and restorative of the entire digestive system. The griping tendency is diminished by the addition of powdered ginger. As heat destroy the properties of this herb it should be prepared as a cold water infusion steeping the pods or leaves for a minimum of 4 hours.

Uses - Treatment of constipation.

Dose - 24 large senna pods for cows. Soak in cold water for a minimum of 4 hours but preferably 7 hours. Add half a teaspoon of ginger to 20 to 24. Give the dose last thing at night at least 2 hours after food has been taken.

Tansy

Actions - Digestive bitter, carminative, emmenagogue, vermifuge, anthelmintic.

Cows and sheep eat the herb, powerful worm expellant, effective against round worm and thread worm and may be used in children as a enema, as a bitter it will stimulate the digestive process, eases dyspepsia, stimulate menses.

Uses - Treatment of all types of worms, debility, causes abortion.

Caution - Avoid during Pregnancy.

Tea Tree Oil

Australian Tea Tree Oil is one of the world's best antiseptics and is also anti-bacterial, anti-fungal and anti-viral which means you can use it with good results on virtually any wound on the skin.

Use for external applications.

Thyme

Actions - Carminative, antimicrobial, antispasmodic, expectorant, astringent, anthelmintic.

Eaten by sheep and goats and is a milk tonic for them, the whole herb is tonic and antiseptic, A favorite Bee herb and should be planted by all apiaries, can be used for digestive or respiratory infections, use as a gargle for laryngitis or tonsillitis, eases sore throats and coughs, bronchitis, whooping cough, asthma, diarrhea and dyspepsia and sluggish digestion,

Uses - Treatment of all digestive complaints including colic, inflammation of the liver, rickets, all pectoral ailments, hysteria, nervousness, sciatica, retention of afterbirth, inflamed or diseased uterus, metritis, worms including hook worm.

Valerian

Actions - Sedative, antispasmodic, hypnotic, hypotensive, carminative.

A powerful nervine and sedative stronger than other herbal sedatives, pain reliever, reduces anxiety, hysteria, soothes the nervous system, reduces high blood pressure, slows and strengthens the heart and calms palpitations, useful for muscle spasms, arthritic pain, spinal injuries, aids indigestion and gas, insomnia, cramps, colic, can help with migraines. Valerian root is one of the most widely used herbal nervines for calming horses as it can relieve anxiety and excitability without reducing the horse's mental faculties or their physical ability to perform.

Uses - Treatment of epilepsy, hysteria, acute constipation, worms, malaria, pain and for sensitive nervous animals.

Externally - The oil is used as a rub for paralyzed limbs, cramps, swollen arteries and veins.

Caution - Do not mix with drug tranquillizers.

Vervain

Actions - Nerve tonic, hepatic, sedative, antispasmodic, diaphoretic. A favorite of Hippocrates, valuable in every type of fever use in the early stages, nervous disorders, eye problems, plague remedy of ancient times, strengthens the nervous system while relaxing any tension or stress, depression especially if it comes on after a illness, seizures, hysteria, inflammation of the gallbladder, jaundice, use as a mouth wash in gum disease.

Uses - Treatments of all fevers, fits, convulsions, hysteria, liver complaints, gallstones.

Externally - Weak and inflamed eyes, inflamed throats, sore and ulcerated mouths.

Wild Yam

Actions - Antispasmodic, anti-inflammatory, anti-rheumatic,
The first birth control pills were once based on this remedy. Used for severe digestive pain in conditions such as colic, dysmenorrhea, and ovarian and uterine pains. Also used in the treatment of rheumatoid arthritis especially when there is painful inflammation. Muscle cramps and spasms, nerve pains and threatened miscarriage.

Dose - For horses 1 tablespoon of powder twice daily.

Willow Bark (White Willow)

Actions - Febrifuge ,bitter tonic, astringent, antiseptic, analgesic, anti-inflammatory, anti-rheumatic.

Willow Bark can be thought of as caveman's Aspirin as it was developed from this. Cattle and horses eat the young shoots and foliage. It is a refrigerant herb valuable in fevers and pain relief but can take a while to get into the system so think of looking for results especially in pain in about a day's time.

Uses - Treatment of all fevers, debility, enteritis, colic, pleurisy, rheumatism, sciatica and urinary infections as the excretion of salicylic acid in urine soothes a inflamed tract.

Externally - Rickets and cramp.

Witch Hazel

Actions - Astringent one of the most widely used ones. Antiseptic.

As with all astringents this herb may be used wherever there is bleeding both externally and internally, commonly used for piles, bruises and inflamed swellings, varicose veins, diarrhea.

Uses - Internally to heal ulcerated and burnt tissues in cases of poisoning, stomach and intestinal ulcers, Externally - wounds, sores, bruises, ulcers, inflammation of the organs of reproduction, torn udders resulting in milk leakage, inflamed udders and glands, sore eyes and inflamed ears.

Withania (Ashwagandha)

Actions - Adaptogen, analgesic, anti-tumor, hormone regulator, pregnancy tonic, rejuvinative.

This herb is a pregnancy tonic for both the foetus and a weak mother, relieves pain by lowering serotonin levels which contribute to the sensitivity of pain receptors in the body. Good for debility, nervous exhaustion especially due to stress and chronic diseases especially those marked by inflammation. Retards various aspects of the aging process and increases stamina and also sexual desire.

Wood Betony

Actions - Alterative, analgesic, antispasmodic, astringent, Bitter tonic, sedative, circulatory stimulant, diuretic.

Juliette de Bairacli Levy says the whole plant possesses a pungent and peculiar aroma especially when trampled on. This would show the plant to have a high oil content. Was once used as a smoke and snuff to treat headaches. Wood Betony is used for severe pains in the face and head consider it for horses with severe sinus or those who always toss there head.

Uses - Treatment of debility, gastritis, diarrhea, acidity, glandular deficiency, arthritis, rheumatism, exhaustion, sciatica, hypertension, kidney dysfunction.

Externally - arthritis, rheumatism, sciatica, rickets, tumors, swellings, boils, abscesses, corns, warts and blisters, gingivitis, as a poultice to draw out splinters and boils.

Wormwood

Actions - Bitter tonic, carminative, anthelmintic, anti-inflammatory.
The foliage is eaten by horses, cows and sheep. Its chief merits are worm expellant (round worm and pinworm) and tonic. A important herb for female ailments, protects against contagious diseases and plagues, insecticide, hair tonic, as a bitter it stimulates the digestive process, fevers, infections.

Uses - Treatment of all worms, failing appetite, gastritis, gastric ulcers, acidity, enteritis, constipation, jaundice, TB, tumor, pneumonia, pleurisy, all female ailments and bladder problems.

Externally - Prevention of falling hair, insecticide especially lice, sores, mange, inflammation of the ear, conjunctivitis.

Yarrow

Actions - Diaphoretic, astringent, diuretic, antiseptic, hypotensive.
It is a famed wound herb for staunching excess bleeding and derives its name from the Greek Warrior Achilles who healed his wounds and those of his soldiers with yarrow blossoms.
The herb is one of the best diaphoretics known to herbalists opening the skin pores and inducing lavish perspiration, sheep seek out the herb on dry ground as a food tonic, fevers, as a urinary antiseptic it can be used for cystitis, specific in thrombotic conditions associated

with high blood pressure.

Uses - Treatment of all fevers, pneumonia, pleurisy, inflamed throat, hemorrhages, uterine hemorrhages, dysentery, hysteria, epilepsy, rheumatism, colic.

Externally - Wounds, skin eruptions, abscess, earache.

Yellow Dock

Actions - Alterative, Cholagogue, purgative, mild astringent.

A powerful blood purifier and astringent. It is used in treating all diseases of the blood and skin. Very high in iron, making it useful for treating anemia. It nourishes and detoxifies the liver and cleanses and enriches the blood.

Used extensively for skin complaints such as psoriasis, a mild acting remedy for the relief of constipation, has a action on the gallbladder.

Uses - Constipation, skin problems, gallbladder problems, jaundice.

Dose - For horses 1 tablespoon of powder twice daily, less if purgative action is too much.

Yucca

Actions - Alterative, anti-inflammatory, anti-rheumatic, laxative.

This herb is gaining attention for its treatment in dogs for arthritis, hip displasia and other degenerative hip and bone diseases. It seems to have a natural anti-inflammatory effect on the body. The saponins in Yucca mimic the structure and effects of cortisone.

Also aids in digestion and is a blood cleanser. Is now being used for gout.

Cautions - Use only the dried root. Long time use may impair the assimilation of the fat soluble vitamins.

Homeopathic Supplement

Homeopathy has been around now for hundreds of years and unlike most other forms of medicine its rules have not changed and will not for they are based on an essential truth. The main rule is Like cures Like or if we break down the word Homeopathy homo means the same and pathy means disease. As Homoeopathy is a very hard science to learn and as it kind of sits or balances on the border of hard science and metaphysics I will not try to explain to you what it is here as it would probably take a whole book to do this but I will say this, in the UK and a lot of countries in Europe it is on and paid for by the National Health System and anything that can get a politician to open their purse must work.

It is said that Homeopathy sits on a three legged stool. What this means is that if a remedy has at least three symptoms in the same strength as the symptoms you are trying to match then that remedy is a potential cure for your condition or if not cure it will offer the condition relief. The more symptoms you can match to the remedy the better the remedy will work for the rule is likes cure likes not vaguely similar cures. Listed below are some common Homoeopathic Remedies and some of the symptoms they cover. The idea is to find one remedy that covers most of your symptoms. To make the remedies as closer a match as we can we ask lots of questions like the ones below and after we gather all the answers we have what is called a good Symptom Picture which we then try to match as accurately as we can to a Remedy. Most Homeopathic Materia Medicas are set out to answer the questions listed below with the mind symptoms being the most important. Questions on time, position and temperature are good for making a choice between to very close remedies. The best Materia Medica for the lay person is Boerickes and you should be able to view this on a few Homeopathic websites.

Symptom Guide Questions

1/. Was there a sudden onset of the condition, at what time?

2/. What time of the day does the patient feel either better or worse.

3/. What is the effect of motion? jarring? walking? running?

4/. What is the effect of drinking fluids? warm and or cold drinks?

5/. Is the patient thirsty or not at all? sips or gulps?

6/. Is the onset from exertion? overeating? weather changes? emotions?

7/. Mental emotional state of patient?

8/. Better warm room? warm air?

9/. Better cool room? cool open air?

10/. Are the respirations upper chest movements or in the abdomen?

11/. Respirations - dry or wet?

12/. Expectoration - watery or stringy mucous, easy or difficult.

13/. Is there coughing

14/. Position - better or worse from sitting? standing? lying? lying on which side?

15/. Along with the condition is there fever? gas? belching? wind?

Modality - The questions above are covering what the Homoeopaths call modalities which basically mean are covering a condition that makes the patient better or worse. I will list the main Modalities below. The Modalities help us to distinguish which remedy is right for the case especially when we have a group that look as though they may all work which is what I am giving you und the disease heading. Using modalities forces you to think what really is going on, is this the nature of the beast or the nature of the disease.

Time - Better or Worse morning, night, weekly, monthly, seasonally etc.

Motion - Better or Worse first movement, rest, exertion, walking, stretching, rising up etc

Temperature - Better or Worse heat, cold, cold air blowing, sudden change etc.

Body Activity - Better or Worse eating, drinking, urinating, defecating, sleep, coughing etc

Weather - - Better or Worse, damp, sunny, foggy, storms, sudden changes etc.

Senses - Better or Worse - touch, pressure, noise, light, odors etc.

Position - Better or Worse lying, standing, sitting, stretched out, doubled up, right side etc.

Mind - Excitement, anger, fear, stress, better busy, nervous all the time etc.

Now read through all the remedies in the Marteria Medica (Homoeopathic Remedy Reference) and you will notice that most of them have Mind or mental symptoms kind of describing the personalities or moods a good example is Nux Vomica, I think we all know a nasty type of individual that this remedy would be suited to and meaning as though the individual is suited to this remedy then the remedy would have a curative action on them but don't expect it to change the nature of the beast. One of the main rules of Homeopathy is the closer the match of the remedy the higher the Potency you use but if you are not used to Homoeopathy just use the 30C potency and remember what I said about the 3 legged stool. Potency is a measure of strength and depth of action.

Remember as mentioned before Homoeopathy sits on a three legged stool. What this means is that if a remedy has at least three symptoms in the same strength as your symptoms then that remedy is a potential cure.

Note - The best prescribing guide for the layman is **Boerickes Materia Medica With Repertory.**

Another good guide is **The Complete Book Of Homeopathy by Dr Michael Weiner.**

I always buy my books on Homeopathy from India as they are quarter the price and there is always a wide selection. Put B. Jain Publishers into the google search engine go to their web site and check out these books and I am sure you will be pleased with what you find.

Disease Nosodes

Nosodes are remedies made from disease material mainly from the tissues, discharges, exudates, excretions, suppurations or secretions of a infected being. Simply stated a Nosode is a homeopathic remedy prepared from a pathological specimen. Rabies Nosode, for example starts with the saliva of a rabid dog and is then potentized.

Nosodes have many uses and are widely used in homeopathic practice to help limit cases of infectious diseases and to help during the recovery phase of a disease especially the ones that linger and drag on. There are Nosodes for most infectious diseases of animals and humans the use of Nosodes in this way is referred to as isopathy rather than Homoeopathy. They are often used in farm situations, to limit the spread and the effects of infectious diseases. This has especially been used as a vital component of mastitis control on many farms, both organic and conventional. One documented event about Nosodes dates back to Napoleon marching his Legions through Europe and spreading Typhoid in their wake, the towns that had the best cure rates were the ones where the local Homoeopaths used a Nosode of the disease.

Nosodes can be used in the prevention of infectious diseases in the manner of vaccination but they work by a completely different mechanism then from the raising of antibodies that vaccines work by. As yet it is not actually known how they work but they have survived hundreds of years ridicule by producing results and will carry on doing so.

The best known study into Nosodes was done by Dr. Christopher Day of England involving 'kennel cough' in a boarding kennel. At the time he was called in, there were 40 dogs in the kennel with 35 that had kennel cough. About half had been vaccinated for this malady. He gave a Nosode to all the animals that were there and all the dogs that came in through the rest of the summer, which was another 214 dogs. He successfully reduced the incidence of kennel cough from over 90% to less than 2%.

Nosodes used for the prevention of diseases are usually given in the 30C potency. A good dosing regime is one dose given night and morning for 3 days followed by one per month for the next 6 months. This generally provides a good level of protection after the first week. A good example of how this can be used is a puppy given the Nosode of Parvovirus at 3 to 4 weeks of age instead of having to wait for 9 weeks for the vaccination, this way the puppy is protected before given the vaccination.

Nosodes can have homeopathic therapeutic properties in their own right. Such Nosodes are found in the Homoeopathic Materia Medica and have undergone a proper 'proving'. Examples are Bacillinum,

Carcinosinum, Medorrhinum, Psorinum, Tuberculinum.

Dose - Dr. Surjit S. Makker recommends 20ml of remedy mixed with 8 liters of water for 100 birds. This medicated water should be shaken well and put in drinkers accordingly. For individual birds give them 2-3 pellets by mouth and keep them calm.

Materia Medica

Note - All Homeopathic Remedies are given in Potency and not in material Form.

Aconite

Characteristics - Aconite is best used in the first stages of a illness, especially when fear and anxiety are present. Symptoms appear suddenly, without warning and they may be caused by exposure to cold winds or draughts or by a severe fright. Symptoms are a marked restlessness, animal displays extreme anxiety or fear, high fever with a burning skin, extreme sweating and a burning thirst, a hoarse dry painful cough, bright light noises stress and cold worsen the symptoms, rest and quiet relieves the symptoms. The pains of Aconite are unbearable, sharp, shooting, burning pains, tingling and numbness. A remedy for fevers and inflammatory states, use at the first sign of all fevers, shivering with cold sweats, difficult breathing, animal shows desire for large quantities of water, symptoms worse at midnight, symptoms improve in the open air.

Mind - Great fear, anxiety, restlessness, extreme sensitivity to pain, worry, foreboding.

Better - In open air, warmth, rest.

Worse - In the evening and night, particularly before midnight, lying on affected side.

Allium Cepa

Characteristics - Increased secretions from the eyes and nose, like those of the common cold. Frequent sneezing with watery discharge which burns the nose and upper lip, but the eye discharge is bland and doesn't burn (the opposite of Euphrasia). Tickling in the throat with incessant cough (feels as if larynx is split) holds throat when coughing. Being in cool open air relieves the symptoms, eyelids are swollen and red, abdominal tympany with wind, this remedy is indicated in the early stages of most catarrhal conditions, mild forms of cat flu can be cut short if given early.

Better - Cold room (except cough), open air.

Worse - Evening, warm room, odors.

Antimonium Tartaricum - Ant Tart

Characteristics - Is characterized by a loose rattling unproductive cough such as is often herd in cats. Respiration can be very difficult with much gasping. There is usually thirst for little and often. Symptoms are worse in the evening, lying down and in cold damp weather or a warm room. Confined largely to respiratory diseases, abundant bronchial secretions, great rattling of mucous with little expectoration, drowsiness, debility and sweat.

Mind - Drowsy and despondent, fear of being alone, child will not be touched without whining.

Better - Sitting erect, from burping and expectoration.

Worse - Evenings, lying down, damp cold weather.

Apis

Characteristics - Apis is used for various types of swelling and inflammation such as that from animal bites and bites and stings from insects, it is also used for measles, mumps, sore throats, sore red eyes and fever. Apis is a quick acting remedy for inflammations especially those ones with edema and lots of swelling which is its main use. Acute nephritis with scanty and burning urine there may be some blood in the urine. . Symptoms are swelling with edema which makes the effected parts look shiny, red and puffy, the swollen parts feel soggy and waterlogged, a fever that develops rapidly but without thirst, extreme restlessness and fidgeting, an irritable nature and perhaps jealous, cool air and cold compresses relieve the symptoms. Pains are burning and stinging, arthritis with swelling, animals seek cold surface to lie on, swollen eyelids, may be swollen ears, may be blood in the urine, in the horse and cow there may be edema in the lower limbs while in dogs abdominal dropsy is seen. Symptoms get worse from heat and improve in the open air and from cold bathing.

Mind - Apathy, indifference, awkward.

Better - By cold, (room, air or application)

Worse - From warmth, pressure, late in the afternoon, from sleeping.

Arnica

Characteristics - Bruises and similar injuries where the skin is unbroken and there is mental or emotional shock. Symptoms are any type of bruising or similar injury caused by crushing, squeezing or wrenching, muscles strains which feel sore and bruised, shock after accidents, there is a fear of being touched because of the pain, good for the soreness after birth and medical operations.

Arnica can be used in potency and also as a cream. The cream must not be used on broken skin or wounds. Animal shrinks away when you try to touch it, symptoms improve when lying down.

Mind - Fears touch or approach, whole body oversensitive.

Better - Lying down or with head low.

Worse - Least touch, motion, damp and cold.

Arsenic Album

Characteristics - Burning pains relieved by heat, anxious, restless, weak and chilly with an air of fear and hopelessness. Anxiety or restlessness are often present where this remedy is indicated. Discharge from eyes and nose are watery and acrid causing ulceration in those regions. The mouth is usually dry and the patient is usually thirsty. Dramatic vomiting and diarrhea often simultaneously indicate its use if the modalities agree. The patient may have wheezing respiration and allergic asthmatic conditions can respond well. The skin can be dry, scaly and scruffy. Symptoms are worse for cold and wet better for warmth. Tries to find relief in motion but immediately feels weak with movement. Restless, feels cold, complains of general weakness, discharges burn the skin.

Mind - Fear with despair and restlessness.

Better - Warmth, open air, relieved by sweat, hot drinks, lying down (but restless).

Worse - Cold air, after midnight eg 1 to 3am. Wet damp weather and near sea shore.

Belladonna

Characteristics - This is one of the great fever remedies, conditions requiring its use usually being of violent and sudden onset. Heat, redness, pain and swelling characterize its symptoms. It is one of the main remedies used in convulsions. Pupils are usually dilated which is a keynote for this remedy. Acute ear inflammation where there is heat, pain and swelling respond well. The mouth is usually dry and there is great thirst. With Belladonna always think BIRDS. B for burning, I for irritability, R for redness, D for delirium and S for spasms.

Mind - Hallucinations, delirium, rages, bites, strikes, desire to escape.

Better - For quiet, dark, rest with slight warmth.

Worse - For noise, touch or jarring motion.

Bellis Perennis

Characteristics - Trauma to abdomen and pelvic organs especially after surgery and child birth if arnica does not give relief. Injuries to the nerves with intense soreness, back ache from hard physical work such as gardening, pain is bruised sore and aching, better cold presses, worse touch, after getting wet.

The animal is unwilling to move and when made to do so evidences pain, muscular stiffness is prominent.

Worse - Left side and cold wind.

Bryonia

Characteristics - This remedy shows both diarrhea and constipation symptoms, the latter usually in chronic conditions. The mouth is often dry and there is great thirst. The tongue is often coated yellow. It is of great help in many cases of rheumatism or arthritis where the symptoms agree. There is often respiratory signs with a hoarse hacking cough. All symptoms are worse for movement and better for rest.

Mind - Irritable, delirium.

Better - Lying on the painful side, pressure, rest and cold things.

Worse - Warmth, motion, morning, eating and touch.

Calendula

Characteristics - The part used is the Flowers and it is used for wounds and skin irritations, it is healing, soothing, anti-inflammatory, astringent, anti-fungal and anti-microbial.

Use as a lotion for cuts, grazes, infected sores, fungal infections, any skin inflammations, regulates the oil production of the skin so is good for acne, to stop bleeding, for bruises and sprains, skin ulcers and minor burns and scolds.

Note - The tincture of this is used as a lotion diluted at 1 to 10.

Cantharis

Characteristics - Important first aid remedy for minor burns and for other pains that feel burning and fiery, also has a healing effect on the bladder, urethra and other parts of the urinary tract where burning pain is the key symptom, burns and scalds especially where blistering and inflammation occur, sunburn, insect bites that feel hot and burn, cystitis. Pains are violent burning, cutting, stabbing or smarting, rawness, use when the animal appears distressed when passing urine, or tries to pass and cannot. Better from warmth rest and rubbing.

Mind - Furious delirium, acute mania generally of a sexual type, crying, barking.

Better - From rubbing

Worse - From touch or approach, from urinating, from drinking cold water.

Carbo Vegetabilis

Characteristics - Patient exhibits mental and physical sluggishness and symptoms come on slowly, generalized weakness of all functions especially digestion, overweight, torpid, lazy, complaints of coldness, pains usually described as burning, pressing pains, wishes to be fanned, digestive problems such as belching often accompany any illness.

Mind - Aversion to darkness, sudden loss of memory.

Better - Being fanned, passing gas, rest.

Worse - Morning and evening, exertion, cold, tight clothes at abdomen.

Causticum

Characteristics - Burns and burning pains such as cystitis also used for dry coughs, burns to the skin especially with marked inflammation and blistering, coughs, laryngitis and hoarseness from straining and over using voice, cystitis especially with involuntary passing of urine when coughing, chronic cystitis, exposure to cold dry air may make symptoms worse.

Mind - Least thing makes it cry, sad, hopeless. Ailments from long lasting grief.

Better - In damp wet weather, warmth.

Worse - Cold winds.

Euphrasia

Characteristics - Affects the mucous membranes of the eyes, nose and chest producing copious watery secretions,eye secretions cause smarting of the skin while the nose discharge is bland. Used for conjunctivitis, eye strain generally but especially from computers, eyes that feel sore and inflamed and look red, hay fever symptoms including a tickly throat, sneezing, a runny nose, and itchy red watering eyes. Sunlight wind and warmth worsen the symptoms. Use for Dogs who have had their head out of the window for too long, symptoms better in dim light or darkness, in all species a tendency to diarrhea occurs.

Better - In the dark

Worse - From light, indoors, in the evening.

Hypericum

Characteristics - Used for bruises and other injuries especially to nerve rich areas like the fingers, lips, ears, eyes ,tail bone, good for the pain of puncture wounds of any cause eg animal or insect. Helps with the pains after operations especially amputations. Pains are violent shooting pains along a nerve path, burning, tingling and numbness. Worse from shock and touch and better from rubbing, horse fly bites, symptoms worse cold better warmth.

Mind - Anxiety, melancholy, effects of shock.

Better - Bending head backward.

Worse - Cold, dampness and touch.

Ipecac

Characteristics - Indicated for complaints of persistent nausea not relieved by vomiting, ailments caused by eating rich or indigestible type of foods such as ice-cream, sweets etc., useful to stop bleeding if blood is bright red.

Mind - Easily irritated, child cries or screams continuously, wanting something but not sure what they desire, holds everything in contempt.

Worse - Warm, moist weather, lying down.

Kali Bichromicum

Characteristics - Has a affinity for the mucous membranes of the body, tough stringy viscid secretions sometimes forming thick yellow green mucous, sinus infections, suited for fleshy fat light complexioned people, general weakness.

Better - Heat

Worse - Cold, beer, morning, undressing.

Kali Carbonicum

Characteristics - Has a affinity for the mucous membranes digestive and respiratory, very tired, anemic, flabby tissues which may be swollen, sweat, backache, weakness, many conditions have a aggravation at 2am to 4am, often stays immobile when ill.

Mind - Very irritable, hypersensitive to pain, despondent.

Better - During the day, sitting down, bending forward, warmth.

Worse - Cold weather, between 2am and 4am.

Lachesis

Characteristics - Many symptoms tend to be left sided, cannot bear tight clothing, symptoms worse on awakening, symptoms relieved with onset of the menstrual flow. Short dry cough, feels relief after coughing up watery phlegm, feeling of constriction in throat and chest, better bending forward.

Mind - Overly talkative, impatient, sad, jealous, no desire to mix with world.

Better - Release of pressure, eating fruit, cold, discharges.

Worse - Pressure, touch, after sleep, heat, hot weather.

Ledum

Characteristics - Has a action on the capillaries and is useful for cleaning up bruises especially around the eyes, mainly used for puncture wounds made by sharp points such as nails and wood splinters and insect bites and stings especially ones that don't heal properly and look blue and puffy. Wounds that feel cold to the touch, septic conditions, sprains, pains are throbbing, tearing ,prickling, they shoot upwards, stiff and sore. Better cold, cold bathing. This remedy was used in the past along with hypericum to ward off tetanus especially in deep wounds

Better - From cold.

Worse - At night and from heat.

Lycopodium

Characteristics - Exerts most of its effects on the digestive organs, liver, kidneys and respiratory systems. The patient dislikes being left alone and appears apprehensive. The nose is often blocked and there may be blisters on the tongue. Eating a little food always satisfies the appetite but appetite is very marked. The belly is usually bloated. The stool appears hard and small and is expelled only with difficulty accompanied by ineffectual straining. Urination is also a slow process and the urine has a red sediment. Symptoms are worse for heat generally and better for cold.

Mind - Melancholy, afraid to be alone, apprehensive.

Better - By motion, on getting cold.

Worse - From heat.

Natrum Sulphuricum

Characteristics - A good liver remedy, emotional and mental difficulties arising after head injury, useful in problems associated with rainy weather and dampness, patient feels every change from dry to wet weather, may remove excess water and fluid retention from the body.

Mind - Lively music saddens, melancholy, inability to think, dislikes to speak or be spoken to.

Better - Dry weather and environments, pressure, change of position.

Worse - Damp weather, damp basements, lying on left side.

Nux Vom

Characteristics - The remedy for overindulgence, adapted especially to thin irritable energetic people who attend with great detail to tasks, quarrelsome, nervous, intelligent, hypochondriacal, oversensitive to noise music and light, craves stimulants.

Primarily used in the digestive sphere, its greatest reputation is in helping disturbances following overeating of unsuitable foods. Feces is usually hard but diarrhea can follow overeating. There is abdominal discomfort, flatulence, irritability and sensitivity to noise. Symptoms are generally worse for noise and better after rest or for damp weather.

Mind - Very irritable, sensitive to all impressions, malicious, disposed to reproach others.

Better - Wet weather, lying down, uninterrupted nap.

Worse - Overeating, mental over exertion, sensory stimulation ie sound, sight, touch etc.

Phosphorus

Characteristics - Irritated and inflamed mucous and serous membranes are the key feature of this remedy. Is a very sudden remedy with suddenness of symptoms. The patient is sensitive to loud and sudden noises (eg thunder fireworks etc). Degenerative processes and bone destruction respond well to Phosphorus. Food is suddenly vomited back up when it has been warmed in the stomach, gums can be ulcerated and bloody. Hepatitis, jaundice, pancreatic disease and nephritis come into its sphere. Urine may be bloody. A very painful cough is also a symptom. Wounds that perpetually bleed may also be helped. The patient is usually in poor body condition. Symptoms are worse for touch, exertion, in the evening and during thunder storm. Better for cold and sleep.

Mind - Low spirits, restless, fidgety.

Better - In the dark, lying on the right side, from the cold, sleep.

Worse - Touch, from exertion and in the evening.

Pulsatilla

Characteristics - Often indicated for those with mild, gentle, timid yielding dispositions who are easily moved to laughter and tears, The Pulsatilla person wants to be held and loved, moods changeable and fickle, the patient is chilly but desires strolling in cold air, symptoms are erratic and change frequently, pains are wandering, pains that grow gradually in intensity, fever without thirst despite dry mouth, bland yellow discharges.

Mind - Weeps easily, timid, fears to be alone - dark - ghosts, likes sympathy and fuss, highly emotional, easily discouraged, sensitive.

Better - Open air, cold applications, consolation relieves symptoms.

Worse - Evening before midnight, warmth, after eating fat rich food.

Rhus Tox

Characteristics - Is the most famous of the rheumatic remedies. The skin and muscular skeletal system are its main spheres. Small red papules in the skin and sometimes vesicles are typical lesions with much scratching. In all cases of damage to muscles think of Rhus and the symptoms of arthritis which are worse after rest particularly if this follows strenuous exertion. The symptoms improve with limbering up , The worst pains are seen as the animal arises from its bed.

Mind - Listless, sad, extreme restlessness, great apprehension at night.

Better - Warmth, walking, from stretching out limbs.

Worse - During sleep, cold wet rainy weather and at night.

Ruta

Characteristics - Has effects on the joints, tendons, cartilages, and the periosteum which is a fine membrane that covers bones and gives it that shiny look, it is also used for eye strain where the vision goes dim.

Used for painful bruises affecting the bones, dislocations, strains to the tendons or joints, aching with restlessness, pains are gnawing, digging, burning, bruised, sore as if beaten, bones as if broken, pain deep in the bones, rheumatism.

Better - From lying and warmth.

Worse - From over exertion, touch, cold wet weather.

Silica

Characteristics - Fits the shy chilly patient who is reluctant to enter the room, chronic inflammatory conditions such as sinus, helps in the removal of foreign bodies such as splinters and seeds, ripens abscesses, ailments attended with pus formation. Use silica and be prepared to use it for a while sometimes up to 3 weeks.

Mind - Faint hearted, anxious, yielding.

Better - Warmth, wet or humid weather.

Worse - Morning, from lying down, cold.

Staphysagria

Characteristics - Suits sensitive people who suppress their feelings and suffer in silence or who boil over with indignation, remedy for cuts and wounds especially those that are from medical procedures and have the mentioned feelings. Nervous states of animals. The pains are stinging, stitching, smarting, squeezing, as if stabbed by a knife. Worse from touch, emotions and suppressed anger.

Better - Warmth, rest at night.

Worse - Touch on affected parts, loss of fluids.

Symphytum

Characteristics - Causes bone to grow and promotes fast healing should be given for all fractures. Used for injuries to the hard parts of the body while arnica is for the soft parts. Also used for eye injuries caused from blows.

Caution - do not use if a pin has been placed in the bone as the pin has to be removed latter.

Tarentula Cubensis

Characteristics - For abscesses, boils, carbuncles, swellings of any kind but especially on the back of the neck where the skin turns black, red/blue or purple with great pain. Deep septic conditions with hardening of the effected part, condition comes on fast, pains are burning, stinging, throbbing, pricking like a needle.

Worse - Night.

Urtica Urens

Characteristics - Can be used for burns and also for cystitis where the urine burns the skin and there is dificulty passing urine. Symptoms are stinging pains, swellings particularly blistery swellings, itching.

Worse - Cool moist air, touch.

Notes

Vitamin C

Vitamin C is the primary antioxidant in the lungs and a powerful antihistamine without side effects. Low vitamin C dramatically increases histamine levels which put you at greater risks for inflammation responses in the body. Always give a high dose of Vitamin C to animals before any operation where they require a anesthetic for the reasons mentioned above as they will recover faster and better from the anesthetic and maybe the inflammation from the surgical incisions will be toned down a bit.

Vitamin C is needed by the immune system and is necessary for healing and the prevention of infections along with being a potent antioxidant with anti-bacterial and antiviral actions. It is also essential for the utilization of the essential amino acids lysine (antiviral) and proline. Another point to consider is that stress depletes the body's supply of Vitamin C so this may be another factor in the cause of many diseases. Vit C is essential for the formation of collagen tissue which is vital in tendons and cartilage so always consider this in muscle and back injuries and especially trauma injuries.

Sodium Ascorbate is good for use on animals as it is virtually tasteless when added to the animal's food and does not curdle milk. This can be used in high doses when needed for example dose till the bowels become loose then back the dose off. For severe situations you can use a injectable Vitamin C, in Australia we use Troys Injectable Vit C which we get from the Agricultural Stock Feed Shops or Co Ops. Use a large gauge needle with this as some animals have rather thick hides and the liquid solution is also fairly thick.

Think of using Vitamin C in all operations and all acute diseases. It is a good last resort to think of before the rifle especially in the deadly acute diseases where as a last resort you would use the injectable form in a intramuscular injection, this can also be a good gauge as to what may happen as these injections hurt like hell so if the animal turns around and gives you a filthy look then there is a good chance that they may live and if they do not seem to notice the injection well the chances don't look too good. So remember always keep a bottle of Injectable C in the fridge for emergencies.

Good Herb Sources Of Vitamin C

Alfalfa, Burdock, Catnip, Cayenne, Chickweed, Dandelion, Hawthorn, Garlic, Horseradish, Kelp, Parsley, Plantain, Papaya, Raspberry, Rosehips, Shepherds Purse, Yellow Dock.

The Safest Essential Oils For Animal Use

Even though there are no specific references to Pigs here this has been included to give you an idea of how you could use oils in the treatment of Pigs. Extreme care must be taken using the Essential Oils on animals. The ones mentioned in these pages seem to be the safest if used in a low dose which is a quarter of what you would use on a human and even this would be too high if used on a mouse so really think about what you are doing and always use a little test dose to check for sensitivity.

Danger - Do not use on **birds** and **cats** as there metabolism cannot handle Essential oils and death will be the most likely result, this includes Eucalyptus and Tea Tree oil.

How Oils Work

Essential Oils work by entering the blood stream via the pores of the skin so the biggest action is on the area applied followed by a systemic action via the blood. The liver is the main blood filter and detoxifier of the body so the liver is responsible for breaking down any drug or blood borne foreigner so with the Essential Oils there is always the chance that if the dose is too high or the application is to frequent the liver may be damaged. Never forget that oils are highly concentrated products. A good example is a budgie, you clipped the wings and one is now bleeding so you put Tea Tree oil on it. Imagine the size of one drop of oil now imagine the size of a Budgies liver and it's fairly obvious what's going to happen.

Below are given the cautions for using oils on dogs, follow these cautions on all animals in general. Most information for these pages was sourced from Kristen Leigh Bells book Holistic Aromatherapy For Animals and Catharine Birds book A Healthy Horse The Natural Way.

Essential Oil Blends

Soothing Skin Essential Oil Blend

15ml base oil of hazel nut or sweet almond oil
2 drops Geranium

6 drops Rosewood

6 drops Lavender

1 drop Roman Chamomile

2 drops Carrot Seed

Combine all ingredients, shake and store in a dark glass bottle. Use 2 to 4 drops of this blend to spot treat small areas of skin.

Mange Treatment Blend

15ml base oil of hazel nut or sweet almond oil

5 drops Lavender

7 drops Niaouli

1 drop Helichrysum

2 drops Sweet Marjoram

After bathing the dog 2 to 4 drops of the blend should be applied to the affected areas twice a day for at least 2 weeks. Observe for a week and repeat if necessary. Try to prevent the dog from licking the area.

Tick Bite Forula

15ml base oil of hazel nut or sweet almond oil

5 drops Thyme Thujanol

3 drops Hyssop Decumbens

8 drops Lavender

For use on bites or immediately after the tick is removed to help prevent infection, reduce redness and inflammation and possibly prevent Lymes disease.

Fresh Breath Oil Blend

5ml base oil of hazel nut or sweet almond oil

6 drops Cardamom

4 drops Coriander Seed

6 drops Peppermint

1 to 3 drops inside of the dog's mouth.

Calm Dog Blend

15ml base oil of hazel nut or sweet almond oil

3 drops Valerian

2 drops Vetiver

4 drops Petitgrain

3 drops Sweet Marjoram

2 drops Sweet Orange

The calming effect ranges from taking the edge off to soothing the dog. Dose is 1 to 6 drops depending on the size of the dog.

Fear or Seperation Anxiety

15ml base oil of hazel nut or sweet almond oil

1 drop Neroli

2 drops Sweet Bazil

4 drops Bergamot

6 drops Petitgrain

1 drop Ylang Ylang

Dose is 1 to 6 drops depending on size of dog.

Flea Free Blend

15ml base oil of hazel nut or sweet almond oil

4 drops Clary Sage

1 drop Citronella

7 drops Peppermint

3 drops Lemon

Store in dark glass bottle. 2 to 4 drops to the neck, chest, legs and tail base of the dog.

Tick Free Blend

15ml base oil of hazel nut or sweet almond oil

2 drops Geranium

2 drops Rosewood

3 drops Lavender

2 drops Myrhh

2 drops Opoponax

1 drop Bay Leaf

Store in dark glass bottle. 2 to 4 drops to the neck, chest, legs and tail base of the dog.

Increasing The Appetite
15ml base oil of hazel nut or sweet almond oil

2 drops Sweet Orange

2 drops Lemon

2 drops Grapefruit

2 drops Lime

2 drops Bergamot

For old and sick dogs this is a gentle appetite stimulant. 2 to 6 drops of the final blend to the neck and chest of the dog gently rubbed in. Repeat as needed up to 6 times per day.

Immune Boosting Blend
15ml base oil of hazel nut or sweet almond oil

2 drops Bay Laurel

2 drops Ravensare

2 drops Palmarosa

2 drops Eucalyptus

2 drops Niaouli

2 drops Coriander Seed

2 drops Thyme Thujanol

2 to 4 drops daily via massage to neck and chest.

Colds and Congestion
15ml base oil of hazel nut or sweet almond oil

5 drops Eucalyptus

5 drops Myrhh

5 drops Ravensare

For relieving nasal congestion or cold symptoms in dogs. 1 to 6 drops rubbed into neck or chest.

Fatigue Blend
15ml base oil of hazel nut or sweet almond oil

7 drops Rosemary

6 drops Tangerine

3 drops Ylang Ylang

Balancing and revitalizing for dogs that are suffering from fatigue and malaise.

2 to 4 drops daily via massage to neck and chest.

Flatulence Blend

15ml base oil of hazel nut or sweet almond oil

3 drops Caraway

3 drops Cardamom

3 drops Cinnamon

3 drops Nutmeg

3 drops Tangerine

1 to 2 drops placed on your dog's food and then 1 or 2 drops given after eating. Many dogs enjoy the taste of this spicy blend and will lick it off your hand. The spice oils of this blend are commonly found in food flavorings so digestion is regarded as safe.

Joint Rub Blend

15ml base oil of hazel nut or sweet almond oil

3 drops Black Pepper

4 drops Peppermint

3 drops Speramint

4 drops Juniper Berry

Good for muscle soreness, arthritis, hip dysplasia and sprains. use 2 to 4 drops of the blend and try to rub in as close to the skin as possible. Do a patch test with this oil as it can be irritating. Patch tests can be done with drop of blend in the arm pit.

Motion Sickness Blend

15ml base oil of hazel nut or sweet almond oil

7 drops Ginger

8 drops Peppermint

Give 3 drops in the mouth

Labor Ease Blend

15ml base oil of hazel nut or sweet almond oil

6 drops Clary Sage

1 drop Neroli

5 drops Petitgrain
2 drops Lavender
1 drop Roman Chamomile
Calming and balancing blend, can be applied to the fur of the neck or chest or 1 to 4 drops can be rubbed in the belly.

Oils For Horses

The safest way to use Essential Oils on your horse are external massage and inhalation. When inhaled the Oil addresses the horses emotional states and stored memories as well as entering the body and having an effect with the most obvious here being Eucalyptus which acts as a bronchodilator (illegal for competition horses in some parts of the US). **Use blends in the same strengths as mentioned in dogs don't go over 2% oil in a blend. Only apply the blends to the affected areas. You can copy some of the dog formulas or make your own using the list of oils.**

Essential Oils For Animal Use

The Essential Oils below are fairly safe for Animal Use

Basil (Sweet) - Helpful for restoring mental balance and clarity. For animals that are suffering nervousness or anxiety, dogs with separation anxiety. Use sparingly (PMC30%). **Horses** - Helps to release most muscle spasms. Used before a event it minimizes the amount of uric acid in the blood and other toxic wastes from exercise. A warming winter oil feeding the muscle fibers and stimulating the blood flow. It is a expectorant removing mucous from a clogged respiratory system when rubbed into the chest and inhaled. Rubbed into the abdomen it may help to relieve the pain and symptoms of colic. May irritate the skin in high doses and don't use in pregnancy.

Bay Leaf - Good for a hair and fur tonic, ticks don't like it, good deodorizer.
Actions - Ant microbial.

Bay Laurel - Used in blends for boosting the immune system especially in dogs. Use only in small amounts in blends.

Bergamot - Combines toning, strengthening and balancing effects with soothing, relaxing and uplifting qualities. Useful for the treatment of fungal conditions such as dog ear infections due to yeast overgrowth. Use in small doses as it can cause photosensitization. **Horse** - Use full for treating any skin complaint especially folliculitis, flaking skin and wounds. Good for lice infections and bites, aids in the healing of any wounds and reduces scar formation. Has a stimulating effect on appetite. Be cautious when applying to the skin of a gray horse or to sensitive skin areas that will be exposed to the sun as this oil can cause photosensitization or pigment changes.

Black Pepper - Warming and circulatory stimulant qualities with low toxicity and irritation. Good for sore muscles, joint pains, arthritis and hip dysplasia. **Horse** - Gives tone to skeletal muscles and warms any winter chills. Dilates local blood vessels and improves local blood flow to the muscles warming the muscles from inside. Arthritic joints respond well to pepper and helps with pain management when used over a long period of time. Strengthens the nervous system. May antidote Homoeopathics.

Caraway Seed - Good for digestive problems, wind, poor appetite, indigestion and bad breath.

Cardamom - Digestive problems, bad breath. **Horse** - Good for treating digestive problems of a nervous origin. Encourages the flow of saliva and good for loss of appetite. It is warming when the body feels cold and useful for easing coughs and respiratory complaints. Highly antiviral and second only to Eucalyptus in that respect. For stallions you can use it as an aphrodisiac. May irritate some sensitive skins.

Carrot Seed - Valuable oil in the use of skin care, dry flaky skin that is sensitive to allergens and prone to infections. **Horses** - Strengthens the mucous membranes so is good for respiratory conditions. Useful for regenerating the skin after wounds or skin diseases and it antiseptic action will deal with minor infections. Has a toning hormone like action that will encourage conception and assist the infertile mare.

Cedarwood Atlas - Gentle stimulating oil that increases circulation and stimulates the release toxins. Good for the skin and fleas don't like it. **Horse** - Sores that are slow to heal, saddle sores, folliculitis etc. and dry flaky skin, encourage the re-growth of coat and adds shine. Has a tonic effect on the kidneys. Dries out excess phlegm and runny noses and removes excess mucous from the respiratory system when inhaled.

Chamomile German - Powerful skin soothing ant inflammatory. Burns, allergic reaction and all types of skin irritations can be quickly calmed with this oil. The oil has a deep blue color.

Chamomile Roman - Valuable for soothing the central nervous system and relieving cramps spasms and muscle pains. It also has analgesic effects which may be used for wounds. In humans this has traditionally been used for teething. **Horse** - The strong analgesic properties relieve dull muscular aches and stubborn spasms. It can also relieve overworked and inflamed muscles. Can be used as a wash to relieve the pain of inflames wounds. Good for calming difficult and unruly horses. Good for unmanageable mares when they cycle.

Cinnamon Leaf - Use the leaf not the bark as the leaf is gentler. Excellent digestive tonic and good for flatulent dogs and is a powerful anti-microbial.

Citronella - Well known insect repeller.

Clary Sage - Sedates the central nervous system, good for calming blends. **Horse** - Has a strong regenerative power where hair loss is involved. Useful on puffy joints caused by long periods of standing. Any swelling in the kidney area caused by strenuous work or sluggish kidney function. Calms underlying tension and soothes anxiety. Useful for a mare having trouble conceiving or nervous of the stallion. Don't use during pregnancy.

Coriander Seed - A toning balancing and strengthening oil that promotes and supports the digestion. It is also a circulatory stimulant and thus a good addition to blends for sore joints, muscles or arthritis.

Eucalyptus Radiata - A well-known remedy for congestion of the respiratory system. The oil has anti-viral, anti-inflammatory and expectorant effects. Can be a flea repellant. Antidotes Homoeopathic remedies. **Horse** - Eases muscular aches and pains caused by over exertion, relieves rheumatic and nerve pains. The anti-viral action is good for respiratory infections and it also soothes the inflammation and reduces excess mucous. Heals sores prone to pus formation. Can be irritating to sensitive skin.

Frankincense - Used to strengthen a weakened immune system and is a good choice for any blend for a sick or elderly animal that needs a systemic boost. Can be used for skin aliments due to its anti-inflammatory and anti-bacterial qualities. Horse - Eases shortness of breath and helps any respiratory problem. Rejuvenating especially for those recovering from a serious injury, tonic for the aging and can be used as a pick me up. Good for stubborn hard to heal wounds. Has the ability to dispel fear and anxiety. Don't use during pregnancy.

Geranium - Has tonic and strong anti-fungal actions, suitable in the use of prevention and treatment of fungal ear infections. Also can be used in tick repellant formulas. **Horse** - Gentle analgesic, has diuretic properties and a tonic action on the liver and kidneys. Balance hormones and emotions so is good for erratic mood swings.

Ginger - Good for the digestive and circulatory systems. Used for motion sickness, sprains, strains and arthritis. **Horse** - Good for conditions caused by cold and dampness. Stimulates circulation to cold joints and is analgesic relieving arthritic and rheumatic pain, muscle spasms and sprains. Is a appetite stimulant and can relieve travel sickness.
Careful on sensitive skins.

Grapefruit - Used for calming, deodorizing and also repelling insects particularly fleas. Has a tonic effect on skin, hair and tissues. Useful for animals with imbalanced sebum production. **Horse** - Gentle effective lymphatic stimulant that nourishes cells while removing toxins. Tonic to the liver. Careful on sensitive skins.

Helichrysum - Actions - Analgesic, anti-inflammatory, regenerative, good for the skin.

Hyssop Decumbens - Different from the normal hyssop. This one is a antiviral and antibacterial and anti-depressant. The oil is also nontoxic and irritating.

Juniper Berry - Stimulating to the circulatory system and good for use in blends used for arthritis and pain. Helpful for balancing oily skin and for acne, eczema and hair loss. **Horse** - Helps stimulate kidney function and this in turn helps to remove metabolic wastes. Don't use during pregnancy.

Labdunum - This oil is antibacterial and astringent. Used for wounds.

Lavender - Antibacterial, antipruritic (anti-itch), powerful regenerative properties. The oil acts as a sedative on the central nervous system. **Horse** - Is cell regenerating and hastens the healing process. Sedates and soothes any wound or emotion. Helps to dispel gas and eases muscle tightness.

Lemon - Calming, strong antibacterial, deodorizer. **Horse** - Stimulates the body to excrete toxins and wastes via the skin, gently astringent and encourages the movement and release of excess toxins. Supports the liver and kidneys. In the cold season gently addresses runny watery respiratory problems and boosts the immune system. For older horses it can be added to rheumatic blends.

Lemon Grass - Antiviral and has a calming effect. **Horse** - Relieves pain in aching muscles and makes the muscles supple. Careful on sensitive skin and around wounds.

Mandarin Green - Good for calming fear, anxiety or stress. **Horse** - Nourishes the peripheral circulation feeding any extremity that suffers from poor circulation. Helps with muscle spasms.

Marjoram - Calming, spasmolytic, strong antibacterial, bacterial infections, wound care and insect repelling.
Meant to be good for calming over amorous male dogs. **Horse** - Warms cold aching joints, relieves muscle spasms and draws bruising to the surface. Helps with the aches and pain of arthritis and swollen joints in old horses. Can help with travel sickness.

Myrrh - Anti-inflammatory, anti-viral, good for puppy teething, treating irritated or inflamed skin conditions or for adding to immune boosting blends. Good for repelling ticks. **Horse** - Its antiseptic action is useful for deep seated respiratory conditions when inhaled. Can be used in a compress to treat boils, chapped or weeping skin conditions and fungal conditions like ringworm. Has a stimulating toning action on the mares reproductive system. Use only short term and not during pregnancy.

Neroli - Calming, stress reduction, anxiety, used for blend for female dogs in labor to ease pain and stress.

Niaouli - Anti histamine, antibacterial, good for allergies manifesting on the skin as well as first aid. Use for cleaning and for preventing ear infections in dogs.

Nutmeg - Canine flatulence, reduces gas production and aids in indigestion and nausea. Stimulating to the circulatory system.

Sweet Orange - Calming, deodorizing, flea repellant, may help in excess sebum production of the skin.

Palmarosa - Antibacterial, antiviral. **Horse** - Helpful when the body is over heated, encourages cellular regeneration and aid hydration by encouraging the flow of fluids throughout the body. Good for stiff joints and aching back.

Patchouli - Gentle circulatory stimulant for the skin and coat and also acts as a insect repellant. **Horse** - Tissue regenerator that aids in the healing of wounds, may address old scar tissue if applied regularly. Used for treating sores that contain heat a compress will cool the wound and help heal. Helps the skin regain its elasticity. Has diuretic properties.

Peppermint - Stimulates circulation, analgesic, sprains, strains, arthritis, repels fleas, flies, mossies' , itching, car sickness. **Horse** - Peppermint has a cooling and analgesic action on heated local injuries. Can burn sensitive skins. Antidotes Homoeopathics.

Ravensare - Anti viral and antibacterial. For animals with compromised immune systems or for young dogs that are prone to infections.

Rose - Stabilizing to the central nervous system, has a gentle tonifying effect to the skin good for adding to blends for itchy or irritated skin.

Rosemary - The oil is mucolytic acting as a expectorant and also aids in cell regeneration. May help in promoting and maintaining hair growth. **Horse** - Stimulates both the mental and physical body into action, can relieve pain without sedating.

Rosewood - The oil has antiviral and antibacterial properties and ticks are repelled by the scent of it. Good for skin conditions.

Spearmint - Similar actions to peppermint, repels fleas and other insects stimulates circulation to the area it is used.

Spikenarde - Calming and grounding, rejuvenating and regenerating to the skin, good for dogs with skin problems, has a similar range of action as valerian.

Thyme Linalol - Antibacterial, anti-fungal, good for skin problems and not as harsh as thyme.

Thyme Thujanol - Has all the benefits of the above thyme as well as being a immune system stimulant and live detoxifier. Can be used in the prevention of lymes disease applied immediately after a tick bite.

Valerian - Calming and grounding, good for dogs with separation anxiety or who are fearful of loud noises, storms, fireworks or new situations. Good as a tonic for the nervous system.

Vetiver - Used in blends for calming, circulatory tonic and strengthens the immune system. **Horse** - Used to treat aches and pains and is a tonic for most body systems. Used for debilitated and distressed horses.

Ylang Ylang - Deeply calming, used in fatigue blends. **Horses** - Commonly used as a aphrodisiac, has an affinity for the adrenal glands.

Notes

Global Warming Edition
Fire, Heat Stress and Global Warming

As I am writing this during summer in the State of Victoria, Australia in the Countryside, the top of Australia in the Northern Territory has a fire burning which is the size of Spain. It just seems to be getting worse all the time. Australia is notorious for its massive fires and now the severity is getting worse, but luckily over a period of 20 years we have changed our habits and ways of thinking and quite a few times now we have managed to save ourselves when the Authorities were overwhelmed and could not help, or the roads were cut off so they couldn't get there anyway. Most farms big, small or Hobby Farms and even isolated properties now have trailers with a 1000 litre IBC tank hooked up to a pump and hose that can be transported where it is needed. Quite a few times now when the roads are blocked local communities have saved themselves with these trailers and on a lot of occasions some people call their friends for help and to bring their fire trailers over. With mobile phones they have now found that they can organize themselves and get multiple trailers out to deal with spot fires and have the situation under control before the Authorities get there. Now with the technical advancement and the falling of prices for drones you can even have a look at what is happening before you even get there or on your way. As far as I am concerned this is the way it should be and as the situation is only going to continue to get worse more people should start to prepare themselves for the worst. As the conditions get worse across the globe many people in remote areas are going to have to learn to look after themselves for as usual most of the help will go to the cities and large towns, so now is the time to start making your plans.

High Temperature Animal Management Needs Good Planning

You need to develop a plan for days of high to extreme temperatures to ensure that your animals will have sufficient shade and water when needed in extreme weather conditions. Extreme heat causes significant stress for all animals with some suffering more than others, so now is the time to review your planning and farm infrastructure so as to provide shaded areas with good ventilation to maximise heat loss. As a gauge we will use 36 degrees Celsius as our danger mark especially if the heat is dry, if it is humid we can relax a bit, but it's time to get our act together. Managing animals in high temperatures requires good forward planning and keeping an eye on the weather forecasts along with developing a plan for days of high to extreme temperatures is essential in ensuring that your animals will have sufficient shade and water on those very hot days. More shade and water troughs would be a good start along with checking the animals more frequently during the hottest days at the hottest times of the day for signs of heat stress, along with all the water points to ensure animals have access to plenty of clean cool water. Make sure troughs or containers are firmly fixed so they cannot overturn and are clean, well designed and maintained to prevent injuries. Make sure the stock does not have to walk too far for water and that they know where all the water areas are and if you use large concrete troughs these will to help keep the drinking water cool. Extreme heat causes significant stress for all animals and it's up to you to ensure the welfare of your animals is maintained. Animals need to be checked regularly throughout the day for signs of heat stress. Remember with Global Warming there is no such thing as normal weather patterns anymore and it's going to get worse before it gets better, if it ever gets better, but that's up to our Governments and the rich elite of the world which makes it even more depressing.

Heat Shelters for Animals

Animals need shelter during extended periods of extreme temperatures especially the very young or old and animals that are in poor condition or sick. Every farm is different but they are all going to get hit with Climate Change one way or another along with the country areas and their populations, so now is the time to have a good look around and consider improvements and see what there is that's going to give you problems in the future. Walk around the property and try to see what's going to cause you trouble in the middle of summer. Where do I need to put shade, are there any sheltered areas that you could use or fence off in an emergency and may add more trees and shade. Due to storms getting worse it may be time to have another good look at your high ground and figure out how you could use it in a flood and maybe how you could save the water by creating dams or ponds. About 30 years ago I was on a farm built on the side of a hill in the subtropics in Queensland that had a near hit by a cyclone. We had to wait a week before we could get into town, and even then we had to pile everyone onto a truck to get there as a car would have been washed away. Ten years later I was on a farm in South Australia 60 to 70 kilometres North of Adelaide during a drought and they stopped us from using the slasher on the back of the tractor, as when the slasher hit a rock the spark off the blade would cause a fire. To be honest I am glad my times nearly up as the future is not really looking all that bright and the reality is that it's up to you now to look after and protect you and yours with maybe a little help from your friends. Now let's have a good look at what's out there to keep your animals cool and healthy in the heat to come. **The best type of shelter during extreme heat should protect the animals from the sun and allow for the cooling effect of wind.** Don't forget to put some water close by. Pets and small animals should be moved to cool areas of the house or a shed.

1/. **Shade Sails** - My favourite and the easiest and cheapest to do is the Shade Sails. These are easy to set up and can be used as a large or small scale setup, or just in the places where you need them. The simplest is the sail on three posts. The best ways to use these are to find the areas on your property with a bit of natural shade and see how much you can increase it using a simple cheap sail with 3 posts. A good and natural spot to choose would be where a stream is in a valley where the animals would head to naturally or any other area in your land that has a natural shelter or one that could be made easily. On different farms I have noticed that animals tend to hang out in certain areas when they rest so this may be a good spot. Another advantage is that you can easily take the shade down for winter so it doesn't have to wear out fast. Shade sails are about the fastest, cheapest and easiest way to go and are a good first choice with fast results.

2/. **Trees and Shelter Belts** – Lots of farms have these; usually they are in an area where it was not worth the effort to get rid of them or too hard to access, or even a danger to the livestock. Maybe it's time these areas are re-examined again to see if they can be used fully or partly as a Heat Refuge. While you are doing this also consider where you could place new trees with large canopies that are fast growing and native to you area. Also consider placing one of these trees beside each water trough to slow down the evaporation rate. Shelterbelts or Hedges are a good idea and can be as big and complex as your imagination. Always have them crossing the farm going East to West so when the sun rises in the east the animals can use the shade on the west and the opposite in the afternoon, so that leaves us with only the mid-day sun to sort out. Always remember to leave regular gaps in the belts and hedges so animals can pass through them easily but also more importantly to allow a breeze to blow through the gaps to help cool the animals. Trees have a cooling effect due to absorption of heat by the leaves. Always check out the fodder trees that can be grown or even better are native to your area and always try to make everything multi-purpose. For those that are interested in this and want more information find yourself a Permaculture Manual as that will give you all the information you need along with plants you can use as stock feed and trees you can use as what they call Pioneer Plants, which you use to protect and fertilize the tree you want to grow which dies off latter after it has finished its work.

3/. - Placement and Construction of Livestock Sheds – Placement is the first and most important consideration especially for heat, but saying that if you live in a place where they have nasty cold winters and lots of snow you will have to decide between which is worse for you and plan accordingly. In winter the sun is low on the horizon so maybe think about making a sleeping and resting area on the longest wall of the structure so as to capture the most heat in winter, then in summer when the sun is above it will run along the roof. Aluminium or galvanised steel are ideal roofs for shelters, kennels, and chicken coops as these materials are very good at reflecting the radiative rays of the sun. Other common construction materials are corrugated iron, timber and shade cloth. You may want to consider having the structures east to west so in summer the sun runs across the roof and maybe insulate the east and west walls. **Outdoor poultry houses** should be positioned in shaded areas away from the sun and in a place where it can get good airflow. Use wide overhangs at the eaves and solid end walls so as to make as much shade as possible. Don't forget that an angled roof will reflect more heat at the hottest time of the day and leave you room for adding insulation in the future if things get worse. Place the nesting boxes in the coolest part of the structure or maybe back to back down the centre as this might be a better place for all the seasons. Again consider insulation on the east and west walls. With any farm construction it is always better to build slightly bigger then smaller as you don't want the risk of animals getting crushed, smothered or injured and always consider the entrance and door sizes as again it's better to make them bigger and avoid future problems.

Heat Stress Tolerances for livestock

Animals at high risk of heat stress are the young, black and dark coloured animals and animals that have been housed and not usually out in the sun with fair skin such as pigs. As always the sun will make it worse for the sick and injured of all kinds and greatly increase the rate of water needed. Heat stress tolerances also vary between different species and different places where animals are farmed so we need to know what's happening in our own area, and how it is going to affect the livestock and what the future outlook may be, as there is no going back now. Your area may not be suitable anymore, or another breed of the same species might be happier in your area. Better to make the decisions sooner than later as it will be far cheaper in the long run. In Australia I was on a farm up North in the subtropics so we got Anglo-Nubian Goats who handled the temperature a lot better than us and most of the other animals and as an added bonus we found them to be highly intelligent. Next we will take a look at how heat stress affects our main animals.

Handling Hot Days and Transport Animals

Try to do all the animal work in the cool of the mornings or the evenings. It is not good for you or the animals to work in extreme heat unless absolutely necessary or in an emergency such as a fire. Some of the farms I have worked on in very hot areas we worked from 6am to 10am and then 2pm to 6pm, which made life more bearably for both the human and the animals. For cattle research has shown that movement or handling during hot weather can increase their body temperature by 0.5 to 3.5° C. Increased body temperature or heat stress will cause losses in livestock and impact on their ability to function. Moving animals during cooler hours can decrease the impact of high temperatures, with a good example being a delay in milking by an hour or more in the evenings can result in an increase in production of up to 1.5 litres per day per cow. Transport of animals should be planned so that climatic extremes are avoided and animals are transported during the cooler hours of the day or at night. I know of an example that went really wrong when the driver was doing all the right things, he was carrying chickens from Adelaide to Melbourne which is a distance of 750 kilometres. He was carrying chickens in cages with water on a semi-trailer which they always tarped so as to keep the wind off the chickens, and always drove through the night so there would be no heat stress and always stopped at the half way point to check that everything was fine. In the last part of the trip the tarp ripped on the side close to the back on the trailer and the poor chickens there had to endure 110 Kph winds for a few hours resulting in about a quarter of them were very naked and not happy. Unfortunately the new owner was not very impressed and asked him what the hell did you do to them, which was about the same time as the drivers offsider burst out in hysterical laughter. This was just one of those things, the driver did everything right, he drove in the cool air of night, he only stopped once to check the load and that was just for 5 minutes. The general rules for transporting animals especially sheep and cattle in severe heat conditions are to use the safest and quickest roots, try to do it in one trip so the breeze through the truck keeps the animals cool. If it is necessary to stop, park the vehicle in the shade and at right angles to the wind direction to improve wind flow between animals during hot weather. Keep the duration of stops to a minimum to avoid the build-up of heat while the vehicle is stationary. In extreme heat reduce stocking densities by about 15% so as to encourage more breezes throughout the trailer to keep the animals cool. In some States and especially in the outback you have to have powerful rifles so if you have an accident you can humanly put down those animals that need it.

Heat Stress Effects on Animals

The general signs of heat stress are panting, increased respiration rate, increased water intake, loss of appetite, listlessness or lethargy, increased salivation and in severe cases unconsciousness and the possibility of death. Here we will go through the different animals and see how they handle excessive heat and what we can do to prevent problems. If your animals are showing signs of heat stress you need to cool them down so start with taking them to the shade, with the best areas being were there is a breeze. To add to this you could use a water sprinkler capable of adding a fine misty spray to reduce the heat even further. Do not soak the animals, just a little bit of mist frequently. If animals are too stressed to move, pick them up and move them or provide shade where they are especially for the larger and heavier animals such as cattle. With cattle the easiest solution is to get the truck and use the truck to block the sun then provide water in 20 litre buckets (or whatever you have), encourage them to drink small amounts often as, a large amount may cause shock and death. After that try to find the biggest water mister bottle you can and spray just spray one of them and see how they handle it especially on the legs and feet, don't try to pour a bucket of cold water on them as the shock could be too much, but they may like a big wet towel put over them. **I have decided to start here with Humans because if you don't look after yourself and get it you are not going to be much use to your animals.**

Humans and Heat Stress

If you are have to deal with heat stress in animals then it's time to learn how to treat Humans with the same condition, as you may be the next victim. This condition can sneak up on you without you realizing what is happening especially if the sun is directly on you head. Heat exhaustion is the beginning of the journey towards heat stroke. One of the fastest ways of getting there is wandering around in the sun on a hot sunny day of over 36 degrees Celsius without a hat on in the middle of a cloudless day. This means the sun is right above you and is beginning to cook your brain very fast. You can develop some really weird symptoms fast and need to get out of the sun. Unfortunately I went through this at about 21 and learned my lesson well. Now that the climate is hotter this is a lesson we should all learn especially for our children's sake as they are the ones that are vulnerable now. Start with your basic First Aid. A pre-warning of Heat Stress can be **Heat Cramps** which usually happen when you work outside in the heat and are sweating a lot and you've used up your excess fluid, so the body decides to tell you by starting to cramp.

Signs of heat stress
Excessive sweating and cold, pale, clammy skin.
Headache.
Dizziness and confusion.
Loss of appetite and feeling sick.
Nausea and or vomiting.
Cramps in the arms, legs and stomach.
Fast weak pulse.
Tiredness weakness.
Being thirsty.
Headache.
Fainting.
Decreased Urine Output.

Take this as your warning sign and get rehydrated and have a rest in a shady cool area. Heat cramps are the mildest form of heat related illness. They are painful muscle cramps and spasms caused by your body's loss of salt and fluid due to excessive sweating. Heat cramps can occur during or after intense exercise and can be a symptom of a more serious heat exhaustion. To relieve the cramps drink some water or even better a rehydration solution which should be in every first aid kit and rest in a shaded cooler area and finish the work in a cooler part of the day. Sometimes we can miss out on the cramps and slowly work our way to Heat Exhaustion without releasing till it is too late. Check all the symptoms and start treatment quickly so as to not make the condition worse. The best you can do is get the patient into a cool house with the air-conditioning running and offer them a long cool drink or even better one with a rehydration formula mixed into it and observe the patient and see what happens. Are they over dressed for the conditions? If so suggest to them that they are overdressed for the conditions. If you are worried that the condition is getting worse don't hesitate to call for an ambulance as the phone operators are usually highly trained and can go through the issues with you.

Signs of Heatstroke

Hot, Red, Dry or Damp Skin.

Cessation of sweating.

Body temperature of 38C (104F) or higher.

Fast Strong Pulse.

Decreased urine output.

Rapid and shallow breathing.

Rapid heartbeat.

Elevated or lowered blood pressure.

Confusion and disorientation.

Can be nausea and Dizziness.

Can be seizure.

Fainting - often the first sign in the elderly.

Remove the person from the heat to a cool shady area, if serious especially in the old and young seek emergency help if available. Remove excessive clothing and take note of vital signs such as pulse and temperature and record them along with the worst symptoms. Cool the person with whatever means available but be careful not to shock them, again it's the young and old you have to be very careful with as a shock could be the last straw. Put in a cool tub of water or a cool shower, spray with a garden hose, sponge with cool water, fan while misting with cool water, or place ice packs or cold, wet towels on the person's head, neck, armpits and groin. Was the person just affected by the heat? Or were they working and exerting themselves in the heat? Is it humid weather? Have you been drinking alcohol (dehydration)? When was the last time you had a drink of water? Without a quick response to lower body temperature, heatstroke can cause your brain or other vital organs to swell, possibly resulting in permanent damage which is why this condition is an emergency situation so it is best to get as much information as you can get, especially of any medication they are taking and talk to the emergency services and see what they have to say.

Homoeopathic Remedies For
Heat Stress and Heat Stroke

Below are Homoeopathic Remedies that can be used for Heat Stress and Stroke. These remedies can be used by Humans and Animals. Instead of giving a higher dose when you consider the situation is getting worse it may be better to go to a higher Potency and see what happens. If the situation gets worse which can easily happen in this condition especially in the old and young and you require Ambulance or Medical Treatment, ensure they know the patient has taken Homoeopathic Remedies as the remedies may be masking some of the symptoms. The most important things you can do while waiting medical help is to keep the patient hydrated, cool, comfortable and in a positive mood knowing that help is on the way.

Remedies Heat Exhaustion

China 6C to 30C - Feeling totally wiped out, drained with trembling. Very useful where there has been excessive sweating and severe dehydration is a factor.

Natrum Carb 6C to 30C - A remedy for sunstroke with a headache that feels like a weight on the head. The person may experience weakness and exhaustion and be sensitive to heat. Important Remedy for Sunstroke when the patient is susceptible to changes in temperature. Good for sensitive people who always seem to get headaches from being in the sun. Remedy for debility and exhaustion and headache caused by the sun. Also good for the chronic effects of sun-stroke. Patient may complain of tiredness and extreme weakness due to hot weather. In most cases, the complaints may get worse with a little exertion.

Gelsemium 6C to 30C - Useful for sunstroke with dizziness, heavy eyelids and a headache that starts at the back of the head and radiates forward. The person may feel weak and lethargic and experience trembling. Light headed, droopy, drowsy, thirstless despite the heat. Occasional chills running up and down the spine. Useful in sun-stroke where there is a high temperature with drowsiness and they may feel weak and lethargic and experience trembling, tendency to coma.

Lachesis 6C to 30C - A good remedy for sun-headaches or after being in the sun where there is faintness and dizziness. The key indicator is the person feels worse after a sleep or nap.

Sun (heat) Stroke

Belladonna 6C to 30C - Indicated for sudden, intense symptoms of sunstroke, including high fever, throbbing headache, red face and dilated pupils. The person may be restless, delirious and sensitive to light and noise. Skin is flushed, hot and dry, rapid strong pulse, pupils are fixed and dilated. Headache that is better for dark, silence and rest. The headache can have violent shooting pains in the head which come and go suddenly making the patient cry out. Heat about the head with cold feet. Blood shot eyes and visible throbbing of the carotids. Use for Sunstroke with Congestion of the Head and Face. People needing Belladonna will experience a burning sensation on the face, a severe congestive headache and redness in the eyes. The patient may faint due to weakness. The skin feels hot, red, and dry, and the complaints may aggravate with the least movement.

Gelsemium 6C to 30C - Light headed, droopy, drowsy, thirstless despite the heat. Occasional chills running up and down the spine. Useful in sun-stroke where there is a high temperature with drowsiness or tendency to coma. In Sunstroke when patient feels dull and drowsy. In such cases, there is weakness along with trembling. The patient may feel dizzy and confused. Works well when there is vertigo with a blurring of vision. In most cases, the patient may feel better on lying down.

Glonoine 6C to 30C - Suitable for sunstroke with a severe headache, pulsating or bursting sensation in the head and a feeling of heat in the head. The person may have a flushed face, dilated pupils and experience dizziness or confusion. Throbbing, bursting headache with a hot face and sweaty skin. A great remedy for the effects of sunstroke and congestive headaches. Indicated when the patient has a severe, sudden headache with a throbbing sensation. The patient complains of heaviness in the head, and a feeling that the head is about to burst. In most cases, the pain in the head may get better after sleeping.

Lachesis 6C to 30C - Good remedy for sun-headaches or after being in the sun where there is faintness and dizziness. The key indicator is the person feels worse after a sleep or nap. Lachesis is an important remedy for a patient who gets a pale face and may even faint during

Sunstroke. Nausea and vomiting, along with a cutting and pressing headache, may also occur. The head is very sensitive to touch, and the headache may get worse with a change in weather.

Other Remedies to Consider

Bryonia 6C to 30C - Severe Headache worse for even a slight movement. Remedy to think of when the person has an *intense unquenchable thirst for water.* The person is definitely better for lying completely still and quiet.

Cuprum Met 6C to 30C - First remedy to think of for heat exhaustion if the main symptom is *cramping or the person makes jerking motions of the muscles.* There may also be light-headedness, a rapid pulse and a cold sweat.

Lycopodium 6C to 30C - Heat exhaustion with gastric symptoms - flatulence or a heavy stomach immediately after eating and worse 4 - 8pm. They are generally better for uncovering and getting cooled down.

Natrum Mur 6C to 30C - Good for sunstroke with heat in the head and a red face, nausea and vomiting. A bursting headache or pain like 'tiny hammers' banging. There may be fiery zigzags before the eyes. Very thirsty and a marked desire or aversion to salty food.

BELOW FOR YOUR INTEREST IS THE OPINION OF A MASTER HOMOEOPATH. NOTE ACONITUM THE ONE THAT I AND A LOT OF OTHERS MISSED OUT, THAT'S WHY HE IS A MASTER. THIS IS REPEATED IN THE CATTLE SECTION.

Heat Prostration for Cattle

George MacLeod (McLeod) (1912 – 1995) MRCVS DVSM Veterinary FF. Hom

Sunstroke

Direct rays of the sun on the head may produce dilation of cerebral blood-vessels which in severe cases can cause paralysis. **Symptoms -** Excitement and restlessness are quickly evident and in the less acute case paralysis of certain muscles takes place, finally leading to failure of the respiratory centre.

Homoeopathic Treatment

Aconitum Napellus 12X. This remedy given at once will help calm the animal and reduce excitement. Dose - one every half-hour for four doses.

Beladonna 1M. A most useful remedy for cerebral congestion. Generally there may be visible throbbing of surface vessels, with excitement and dilated pupils. Dose - One every half-hour for four doses. It should be alternated with Aconitum.

Glonoine 30C. One of the main remedies for exposure to sun. The animal exhibits signs of pain in the head, such as throwing the head against any convenient object or banging on the ground. Recumbency is usual with unsteadiness of movement if made to rise. This remedy will do much to reduce the tension in the cerebral blood vessels. Dose - one every hour for four doses.

Heat Exhaustion

Accumulation of body heat may arise after exposure to a long spell of hot weather when the heat builds up in the body. It can be made worse by exercise. Factors which may influence this condition apart from heat are lack of proper oxygenation, fatigue, and insufficient intake of water, together with unnecessary handling, during prolonged hot weather. **Symptoms -** Rapid respirations are a constant sign along with depression and anorexia. The mouth is usually open and frothy mucus accumulates. A rapid pulse is present, while an extremely high temperature is constant. The conjunctivae become congested and motor reflexes are lost.

Homoeopathic Treatment

Glonoine 30C. As Glonoine 30C for Sunstroke.

Natrum Muriaticum 30C. A useful remedy for stabilising the salt metabolism and preventing loss. Dose: one every three hours for four doses.

Sulphur 30C. This remedy is useful for reducing the effects of heat generally, enabling the animal to make a quicker recovery. Dose - one dose every two hours for four

doses. The administration of these remedies will help the action of cold water applications, which are always extremely valuable in reducing heat.

Pigs and Heat Stress

Pigs are going to have a problem with climate change as they are unable to cool themselves with perspiration as humans can do, which makes them very susceptible to heat stress. Another problem is that they also get sunburnt, and should not be exposed to long periods of direct sunlight or extremes of temperature. Problems may begin at about 25 Celsius. Outdoor pigs survive the heat naturally by finding shady cool areas with a breeze and increasing water uptake along with lying on a cool surface. As the heat rises they would then start looking for places where they could make or find some where to make a mud bath, or head off to their local mud bath and have a roll in the mud to cool down with the mud also being their sun tan lotion. Pigs that are being fattened especially in summer can suffer heat stress from about 20 Celsius onwards, remember calories make heat. Signs of heat exhaustion in pigs can include open mouth breathing, panting and making more noise than usual, blotchy skin, stiffness, muscle tremors, and a reluctance to move. They will also reduce the amount of food they are consuming to slow the internal heat that is produced by digestion. When the animal starts panting very hard, that's when you are in trouble, especially if the heats going to last for a long time. A good start would be soaking a big towel with cold water and putting it on the pig's neck and back along with a long cool drink. Always check the young first as they are usually the ones that are affected first and the most, especially if mum stops producing milk, followed by the sows as they have a higher death rate during heat stress. Continuous access to clean water is critical for pig health. The key clinical signs and symptoms include a high respiratory rate, distress and a rectal temperature of 43°C. Part of the problem with pigs is that they don't sweat and they have small lungs so panting may not give much relief.

Symptoms of Heat Stress

Respiration increases and may lead to panting.

Lethargic when moving, slowed down.

Feed intake is slowed so as to reduce internal heat.

Reduced growth in feeder pigs and maybe the young.

Reduced milk production in lactating sows.

General loss in weight.

Diarrhoea.

Increased water consumption.

Increased urine output.

Muscle trembling and weakness.

Transporting Pigs during Hot Days

Hots days are not good for transporting pigs especially when it gets over 25 Celsius. It is best to avoid transporting pigs on hot or humid days. If you have to move them ensure they are transported in a covered and well ventilated trailer to avoid sunburn and to have a cooling breeze. The hotter it gets the more you have to reduce the loading density for example above 25C reduce loading by 10 percent and the hotter it gets consider more so as to allow the pigs to lie on the floor and ensure they are having a good breeze pass through them. On arrival unloaded immediately and give access to cool clean water and shade.

Cattle and Heat Stress

As some places are more affected by climate change then others along with the related water changes due to the changing weather patterns, there will be many changes in the breeds of cattle as their suitability in certain areas becomes questioned. A lot of the British breeds are not going to like the heat and no doubt there will be a lot of experimenting with crossbreeds now and into the near future. Cattle are more prone to heat stress than sheep and goats. Beef cattle with black hair suffer more from direct solar radiation than those with lighter hair, while those with pink skin are at risk of sunburn. Lactating cattle are more susceptible than dry cows because of the additional metabolic heat generated during lactation while high producing dairy cows are more affected by extreme heat than lower producing cows. Heavy cattle over 450kg are more susceptible than lighter ones to sun and heat stroke and no doubt all the overweight ones are.

Symptoms of Heat Stress

Reduced feed intake or change in feeding.
Cattle stand rather than lie down.
Bunching up in shaded areas.
Bunching up around the water trough.
Rapid shallow breathing or open mouth breathing.
Respiration rate increase with the heat.
Panting at higher temperatures.
Increased saliva production.
Lack of coordination and trembling.
Heatwaves can cause rapid dehydration in calves.
Sick or stressed cattle do not like heatwaves.

In regards to heat, cattle and cows do not sweat effectively and rely on respiration to cool themselves. To add to the burden the fermentation process within the rumen creates additional heat which accumulates during the day and dissipates at night when it is cooler. This creates a problem during heatwaves, especially if they last a long time and even worse when the temperatures just keep on going up. Cattles core temperature peaks 2 hours after the peak temperature of the day and then it takes at least 6 hours for their heat load to dissipate. Heavy cattle have a harder time with heat stress due to increased fat deposition and will need more time for recovery. As respiration is used for cooling keep your eyes open for animal's with respiratory problems as they will fare worse and like the canary in the cage they should give you the first warnings of what may come if the temperatures do not drop. Water is the fastest and quickest way for cattle to reduce their core body temperature so you have to ensure that they are able to get it which creates more problems. As we know that the climate is only going to get worse it should now be a priority to add more water troughs and more shady cool areas for stock and allow them the time they need to get used to the changes.

Heat Prostration for Cattle

George MacLeod (McLeod) (1912 – 1995) MRCVS DVSM Veterinary FF. Hom

Sunstroke

Direct rays of the sun on the head may produce dilation of cerebral blood-vessels which in severe cases can cause paralysis. **Symptoms** - Excitement and restlessness are quickly evident and in the less acute case paralysis of certain muscles takes place, finally leading to failure of the respiratory centre.

Homoeopathic Treatment

Aconitum Napellus 12X. This remedy given at once will help calm the animal and reduce excitement. Dose - one every half-hour for four doses.

Beladonna 1M. A most useful remedy for cerebral congestion. Generally there may be visible throbbing of surface vessels, with excitement and dilated pupils. Dose - One every half-hour for four doses. It should be alternated with Aconitum.

Glonoine 30C. One of the main remedies for exposure to sun. The animal exhibits signs of pain in the head, such as throwing the head against any convenient object or banging on the ground. Recumbency is usual with unsteadiness of movement if made to rise. This remedy will do much to reduce the tension in the cerebral blood vessels. Dose - one every hour for four doses.

Heat Exhaustion

Accumulation of body heat may arise after exposure to a long spell of hot weather when the heat builds up in the body. It can be made worse by exercise. Factors which may influence this condition apart from heat are lack of proper oxygenation, fatigue, and insufficient intake of water, together with unnecessary handling, during prolonged hot weather. **Symptoms -** Rapid respirations are a constant sign along with depression and anorexia. The mouth is usually open and frothy mucus accumulates. A rapid pulse is present, while an extremely high temperature is constant. The conjunctivae become congested and motor reflexes are lost.

Homoeopathic Treatment

Glonoine 30C. As Glonoine 30C for Sunstroke.

Natrum Muriaticum 30C. A useful remedy for stabilising the salt metabolism and preventing loss. Dose: one every three hours for four doses.

Sulphur 30C. This remedy is useful for reducing the effects of heat generally, enabling the animal to make a quicker recovery. Dose - one dose every two hours for four doses. The administration of these remedies will help the action of cold water applications, which are always extremely valuable in reducing heat.

Horses and Heat Stress

The best example we can use for Heat Stress is the racing horse. Exercise results in the generation of heat, and in a horse race the horses can produce enough heat to increase the body temperature by one degree Celsius for every minute of the race. For your average non-working horse its problems in climate change could be high temperatures and humidity, lack of wind or air movement in housing along with heat, poor ventilation and dehydration, while outside there would be exposure to direct sunlight and heat with maybe hot dry winds and not much shade. A horse's natural response to heat is usually to increase their sweating along with the rate of breathing and to move more blood into the capillaries under the skin so as to cool it a bit before entering the main blood stream again, that is of course if it didn't have a cold drink of water first.

Symptoms of Heat Stress

Excessive or profuse sweating.

No sweating. (Runout of spare water).

Skin that is dry and hot.

Reduced feed intake.

Rapid shallow breathing or panting.

Flared nostrils.

Unpredictable behaviour and gait.

Very high body temperature.

High respiratory rate.

High heart rate – over 50 beats per minute.

High rectal temperature over 39 degrees Celsius.

A simple test to determine if the horse is dehydrated is to pinch the horse's skin on the neck and see if it resumes its original position immediately, if it takes a while to resume its normal position then it's dehydrated. As usual it is the old and young that can get into difficulties fairly fast so always keep an eye on them when it gets too hot. The very young and foals have a very poor heat regulating ability and can overheat just by standing in the sun so great care is needed for them especially if mum isn't all that bright. It is very worthwhile to have handy a large salt and electrolyte formula that you could use in emergencies, which should be easily found at any good horse shop. Horses that are overweight and not used regularly, along with not being used to hard work are some of the main victims of heat stroke. Horses with difficulty in breathing and looking stressed that develop diarrhoea or signs of colic, or stop sweating are in need of help. Take the horse to a cool and shady area and hose down the horse gently, if you fear the water is to cold sponge the horse down or do a mixture of both. As the horse settles direct the hose to the insides of the legs, head and neck areas following the areas where there are large blood vessels so as to help cool the blood, which in turn will help cool the body internally. Don't forget the wet towel trick especially for the young. Excess water must be scraped off afterwards unless there is a good breeze, as water in the coat on a hot, humid, still day will act as an insulator and it will quickly warm up again. You can use fans to cool and help evaporate the water which will increase the cooling. Offer a bit of water along with water dosed with electrolytes and let them choose which they want but slow them down if they get to greedy. Sometimes it can take an hour or more to get the temperature back to normal. Allow the horse to recover for about 10 days keeping a good eye on them. Restrict exercising your horse to the early morning and the cool of the evening when it is the coolest. If they liked and chose the Electrolytes before you can also add it to their feed regime for a few days to replace essential salts lost through sweating.

Sheep and Heat Stress

Heat stress in sheep is a significant concern, more so in climate change where weather becomes unpredictable, unreliable and extremes become normal. Here the cold breeds will be affected the most as they tend to have shorter bodies and legs, short thick ears and denser fleeces, so these will have a very real risk of fatalities if signs are not recognised early and steps taken to reduce the risks. High temperatures will also affect feed intake, growth rates, fertility, conception rates and are often accompanied by high humidity which makes the situation worse. The hotter the summers get the more the fodder will be affected and to make it worse the rain may change its normal patterns and what may have been good pastures will turn not so good, maybe now is a good time for a rethink and a change in plans. As you know, plenty of fresh cool water is needed to keep sheep healthy and heat stress free, so now is the time to increase the number of troughs and shade so you are prepared for the worst, and save yourself from the problem of all the troughs being over crowed and causing problems. On average sheep will drink one to two gallons (3.7 litres to 7.4) of water a day, with lactating females needing more. Young animals need to drink more often as they have a faster metabolism but only a small tummy.

Symptoms of Heat Stress
Shade seeking.
Crowding at water troughs.
Bunching to seek shade from other sheep.
1/. Open mouth breathing or panting.
2/. Head extended, tongue protruding, profuse salivation.
1 is the beginning, 2 is really bad.

Increased Respiration.
Increased Respiration with deep flank movements.
Wetting head in a water trough.
Weakness or inability to stand.
Rectal temperature above 41°C. (urgent)
Front legs held in a wide stance.

In extreme heat sheep will decrease their grazing time and spend more time in the shade, especially during the heat of the day, and will graze mostly in the evening and early morning hours. If you find heat-stressed animals move them to a cool, shaded area with good air circulation and for those that are in serious trouble with their head extended and tongue protruding it's time to start to lower body temperature. Sheep should be cooled by applying rubbing alcohol to the area between their rear legs as this area is not covered with wool and has a lot of vascular activity which means we will be cooling not only the skin but the blood as well, as it travels back to the heart. Don't accidently set the poor thing on fire by smoking or having it next to an electric fence. For sheep we do not wet the wool areas as this will actually make matters worse as air will not be able to pass through the fleece. With a hose carefully wet the underside and legs avoiding wool areas along with trying to get a breeze flowing in the same area. Work slowly but surely as you do not want to give a stressed animal the shock of a rapid change as that may be the end especially for the old and young. Other cooling treatments include ice applications and cool water enemas, but only do those for the first time with a vet who can show you how to do it properly and what to do if something goes wrong. Always offer heat-stressed sheep ample water and encourage them to drink small amounts and observe how they are handling it. If you have a water misting bottle it makes it easier to cool the legs and belly and any other place where there is no wool.

Goats and Heat Stress

Goats are similar to sheep in heat stress especially the Angora Goats which like sheep have fleece and the problems that go with it, but have an advantage by having horns which can act like a cooling radiator in a car due to the amount of blood supply flowing through the horns. A cold pack wrapped around the horns may help with cooling but not a frozen one as we don't want give them a brain freeze. Other than the Angora, most goats handle the heat far better and a lot of them are breed for the heat such as the Anglo - Nubians who I helped farm in the tropics with their long floppy ears which help in cooling and long legs which keep them high from the grounds radiating heat. Lactating goats require more water in order to produce milk. As usual the very young and the very old goat will be less heat-tolerant, while the darker coloured goats attract more of the sun's heat and can overheat faster than a white goat. Sunburn can be a problem with light-skinned and coloured goats. Heat stress can lead to heat exhaustion or heat stroke. Providing shade and plenty of fresh water help most goat varieties avoid heat stress.

Symptoms of Heat Stress

Shade seeking.
Crowding at water troughs.
Bunching to seek shade.
Open mouth breathing or panting.
The goats become lethargic.
Increased Respiration Rate.
Weakness or inability to stand.
Rectal temperature above 40°C. (urgent)

Similar to Sheep, Goats pant a lot when the weather is hot. If a goat can't stop panting, stops eating and drinking, and can't get up, it is most likely suffering from heat stress. Rectal temperatures over 40 degrees Celsius are a serious threat and cooling will need to be done along with shade, water and a cool area to recover. Non wool goats can be cooled down using water misting bottles or a fine mist hose especially on long floppy ears (be careful not to get water in the ears) and the horns which can act as cooling radiators along with spraying the rest of the body. If the air is not moving then bring out a few fans. Give the Goat access to cool clean water, small amounts regularly. The main method of transferring heat from a goat varies based upon the air temperature and **humidity,** which is the main killer in the equation. Evaporation will remove heat from the goat but it is critical that the humidity not be very high. Evaporation rates are increased when air passing above the coat has a lower humidity.

Dogs and Working Dogs Heat Stress

Dogs don't sweat as humans do instead they release heat by panting and sweating through their paw pads and nose. If they cannot cool themselves their temperature begins to rise. Be aware of how hard your dog is working in the heat, especially when there is High Humidity. If the heat and humidity are high save the work for another day if you can, and always plan your work with the help of the weather forecast. If they must work, it should only be during the cool times of the day, and they must have regular breaks with access to water and shade. Carry water with you if possible and offer small amounts often. Stop work for a dog suspected of suffering from heat stress and check them out and offer water, if you are still worried put them in a water trough and cover their back with water and see how they react. If you are still not happy put them in the shade with a cool breeze if you can.

Symptoms of Heat Stress

Heat stress – Increased thirst and panting

Dry nose (caused by dehydration)

Heat Exhaustion - Heavy Panting and Weakness

Heat Stroke – Drooling, Dizziness, Collapse.

Increased heart rate and breathing

May be vomiting and diarrhoea.

Muscle tremors and seizures.

Collapse.

Ensure your working dogs have access to shade and a source of clear fresh water at all times when they are kennelled or resting. Ice cubes in a dog's water bowl will help to keep water cool. Do not leave dogs tied up on the back of a ute in the sun and on days over 28C dogs must have a layer of insulating material between them and the metal tray. Always park in the shade and provide water and breeze if you can. Do not leave dogs locked in parked cars. Begin treatment for Heatstroke by moving the dog to a cool shaded area, hopefully with a breeze and begin cooling your dog by wetting down their body with a hose or bucket, but avoid the face. I used to start at the back using my hand to push the fur upward and a low pressure hose following and then do the sides. If there is no breeze then get a fan out to make one as we need the evaporation of the water to do the cooling. Keep doing this for a while and they will generally let you know when feeling better. For pets leave them at home during heatwaves as much as possible with plenty of water and shade and do not force the animal to exercise in hot, humid weather. Exercise pets in the cool of the early morning or evening so as to prevent foot burns from the tar on the roads and hot concrete. Because a dog is much closer to the ground hot asphalt and concrete can heat up quickly, and its paws can sustain burns or injuries. Dogs can get sunburned so protect hairless and light-coated dogs with sunscreen when they will be outside in the sun for an extended period of time. Put sunscreen or zinc on exposed areas of pink skin. Animals with long coats can be clipped to increase comfort in hot weather.

Cats and Heat Stress

Heat exhaustion is the prelude to heatstroke, so you have to move fast before the condition deteriorates. Signs to look out for in Cats are restlessness and restless behaviour as they try to find a cool place, which is usually under the house lying on the cool soil and if they are lucky a nice breeze. Other signs are panting, excessive grooming, drooling, pacing up and down and sweaty paws which are all an effort to cool down. Heatstroke occurs in Cats at about 40 degrees Celsius

Symptoms of Heat Stress
Panting or trouble breathing.
Panting increases.
Drooling, restlessness.
Diarrhoea.
Vomiting.
Staggering, Lethargy.
Muscle tremors, Seizures.
Increased Heart rate.
Disorientation.
Red flushed tongue or gums.
Little to no urine, Coma.

Cats that are at high risk of heat stroke are the old and young, those with a health problem, the fat cat and the flat faced breeds such as Persian or Burmese. Cats with long thick coats need to be trimmed before the heat of summer begins. Prevention is the best way to go especially if you know a heatwave is coming, find the coolest area in the house and set the cat up there with plenty of cool water. That should hopefully save them from burning their feet on hot concrete or tar or dehydrating in the hot breeze. Also on the worst hot days consider giving them wet cat food but in smaller amounts spread out during the day as this would take a lot of workload off the digestive system and keep up the hydration. Our old cat that was fairly bright always went under the house in hot weather and cooled herself on the nice cool soil. If you think your cat is suffering from heat stress take them inside to a cool room and have a feel of the floor temperature to see if it is cool. In severe cases where you know the cat is in trouble start with a temperature check which is done rectally with the normal temperature being just slightly over 38 degrees Celsius to 39.2. Temperatures over and above 40 degrees Celsius are a cause of alarm. Provide cool water and encourage them to drink, but not too much at a time. If the cat has had a drink but still looks bad then we have to cool them manually. Find a water bottle that can be used as a mister for spraying and gently and slowly spray the tummy and chest and get a fan set on low speed breezing into the tummy and chest area. If they are not complaining but seem to need more help you can get 2 hand towels and soak them in water and ring them out but not too much, then scruff the towels up and put the first one between the front paws and then point the fan at it but not too close and see what happens. What we are doing is using the evaporation to cool down the cat. If the cat is happy do the same with the rear legs and aim the fan at the middle of the cat. Adding a small amount of rubbing alcohol to the water can also help speed up the evaporation and cooling effect. Check the temperature every 10 minutes so you know what is happening.

Poultry Heat Stress - Chickens

Here we will only deal with chickens as they are the most common small acreage and home reared poultry and are similar to turkeys in heat stress. Ducks and Geese will just take over the swimming pool in a heat wave and probably be happy in a bath tub under a shady tree. Chickens that are too hot will pant and spread their wings to release body heat. Panting releases water into the air which evaporates and helps to cool the chicken, but you can only do that for so long as eventually it will cause dehydration and a pH imbalance. High humidity decreases heat loss from the lungs which makes the birds more prone to heat stress. When the temperature starts to get to hot for chickens they naturally lose heat through their comb, wattles and other areas not covered by feathers and no doubt by a long cool drink. Poultry should not be wet down unless there is a breeze to aid the cooling process and increase air movement around them. This can be done with fans, ventilation, or wind movement. Warm water is less effective for cooling chickens and will cause fungi, mould, bacteria, and other microbes to grow in water which create other problems. You can also add electrolyte solutions to the drinking water in heat waves so as to help prolong the time till dehydration becomes a problem but only do this for no more than 3 days.

Symptoms of Heat Stress

Panting.

Spreading Wings.

Increased thirst.

Lethargy – slowed down.

Decrease in egg laying.

Chickens do not have sweat glands so one of the main ways they try to cool down is by spreading their wings especially when there is a breeze around. If you see them doing this then it's time to get the fan out. Heat stress can cause a decrease in eggs as mentioned before but also dehydration which decreases the water in the egg and electrolytes in the body. Layers can also become calcium deficient which will cause the egg shells to become thinner and weaker. Chickens in heat can also lose weight and become susceptible to other diseases. A good rule of thumb is that when temperatures rise between 24 to 27 degrees C, it is time to check and begin cooling off your chickens. If temperatures are closer to 37 degrees or beyond, it can be dangerous. Always plan for the worst and hope for the best. During a heat wave feed chickens during the early morning or evening, the coolest parts of the day. Remember calories are a measure of heat, food actually makes you hotter. Keeping the coop cool is an excellent way to make sure your flock stays comfortable during hot weather. Regularly clean out litter as a build-up of litter that has started to decay produces heat, so by removing litter you lower the moisture in the coop, which reduces the relative humidity. Make sure your coop has grass around it and not bare dirt as grass absorbs heat, while dirt reflects heat. Always place a coop where there is a breeze as this is the best way to lower heat and keep up the ventilation. Keeping the water where the breeze exits the coops can help in reducing the humidity inside the coops. Air flow removes hot air and humidity. If you cannot get sufficient natural airflow install fans.

Making your Own Fire Trailer

Here we will go back to the beginning. I saw my first Fire Trailer in use in 2006 on a farm I was living on in South Australia 50Ks north of Adelaide City. As it was very hot there was a fire ban. The area around Adelaide is very rocky which makes it very annoying for the farmers. In the early 18th century convicts starting working on the problem by clearing the fields of rocks and using the rocks to fence the paddocks. It was a good idea at the time but in the future it created a problem for tractors using slashers to keep the grass down as the paddocks were littered with small rocks which cause big sparks when the blades hit them which in turn starts fires that can get out of control fast especially if the wind picks up which seems to happen every time you hit a rock. In times of fire danger when you had to use the slasher you would hook up the fire trailer and park it in the middle of the paddock that you were slashing. The fire trailer was mostly made up of bits and pieces found around the farm and put together. The main bed for the equipment was an old 4x6 foot common trailer which had been strengthened on the floor so as to support the 1000 litre IBC tank and light chains each side with large fence strainers to tension the tank to the trailer. The wheels had 4wd tyres that were wider and stronger along with all the wheel bearings being renewed. This trailer had the petrol engine water pump at the front, mounted on the A frame of the trailer with the pump facing the trailer and the pump motor facing the vehicle. The main hose attached to the pump was the red standard fire hose that you would usually see on the walls of government buildings looking like a red circle on the wall with the black thin hose (Red Fire Hose Reel) which you can usually get very cheaply at the local auctions. Some people like the pump and hose at the front of the trailer while other like it at the back of the trailer. The 1000 litre IBC tank is 4 x 4 feet so on a 4 x 6 Trailer you have 2 feet at the back to mount the pump and the hose wheel. Make the mounting for the hose reel very strong so someone standing on the back can support themselves and use a hose at the same time as this is how they commonly put out the reoccurring spot fires with the driver heading to the fires and the person at the back putting them out. The design for your fire trailer is only limited by your imagination and must be set up by you for your own conditions and needs. You could do this as a joint project with your neighbours or other farmers in the area which could save you a lot of money with an example being buying your pump and other equipment in bulk for a discount which has another advantage of many people using the same equipment so they are familiar with it which is very helpful in emergencies. If you have a group networking together you could have a base station that could invest in a few drones that will give you the advantage of where the fires are in your area or when to run away. It's up to your imagination or for some just survival as this has been well and truly proved now and has saved many life's in Australia especially in the hills and ranges where the roads are easily blocked and the only ones that can save you are you and your neighbours. Don't forget fire trailers can also be used for lots of other purposes such as filling up long distance water troughs, mobile cleaning units, mobile cooling units for heat stressed animals or whatever your imagination come up with. We will end by showing you a cheap and basic modern unit designed solely for firefighting.

BASIC - Pull Start - Fire Fighter 1000L Trailer
A$2,241.00

Locally made Australian Galvanised Chassis

1350Kg Axles, Running Gear

Pull start 6.5hp generic engine (Remanufactured)

Up to 60m head (pumping vertically up)

Up to 8m suction (sucking vertically up)

Up to 200 Liters Per Minute

Reconditioned Firex Red Fire Hose Reel

36 Meter 19mm hose with brass twist nozzle

B-Grade Reconditioned IBC 1000 L Tank

Reconditioned Rims and Tyres

Economy clamp on Jockey Wheel

Mudguards

Fittings

https://egritech.square.site

www.ingramcontent.com/pod-product-compliance
Lightning Source LLC
Chambersburg PA
CBHW081100290526
45795CB00006B/1933